Morning Sickness 24/7

Morning Sickness 24/7

◆

Fifty Ways to Help Cope With Hyperemesis Gravidarum

Written by:
Tabby L. Silcott

iUniverse, Inc.
New York Lincoln Shanghai

Morning Sickness 24/7
Fifty Ways to Help Cope With Hyperemesis Gravidarum

Copyright © 2007 by Tabby L. Silcott

All rights reserved. No part of this book may be used or reproduced by any means, graphic, electronic, or mechanical, including photocopying, recording, taping or by any information storage retrieval system without the written permission of the publisher except in the case of brief quotations embodied in critical articles and reviews.

iUniverse books may be ordered through booksellers or by contacting:

iUniverse
2021 Pine Lake Road, Suite 100
Lincoln, NE 68512
www.iuniverse.com
1-800-Authors (1-800-288-4677)

Because of the dynamic nature of the Internet, any Web addresses or links contained in this book may have changed since publication and may no longer be valid.

The information, ideas, and suggestions in this book are not intended as a substitute for professional medical advice. Before following any suggestions contained in this book, you should consult your personal physician. Neither the author nor the publisher shall be liable or responsible for any loss or damage allegedly arising as a consequence of your use or application of any information or suggestions in this book.

ISBN: 978-0-595-44200-3 (pbk)
ISBN: 978-0-595-88531-2 (ebk)

Printed in the United States of America

For Grace

Contents

Acknowledgements xi
CHAPTER 1   Call the Doctor's Office Before you Go 1
CHAPTER 2   Bring someone with you to the appointment 2
CHAPTER 3   Change your doctor if needed 3
CHAPTER 4   Lose the guilt 5
CHAPTER 5   Request time off work if necessary 7
CHAPTER 6   Carry trash bag at all times 8
CHAPTER 7   Get a haircut 10
CHAPTER 8   Hire a babysitter 11
CHAPTER 9   Research 13
CHAPTER 10   Ask for help 15
CHAPTER 11   Ignore others who doubt you're sick 17
CHAPTER 12   Keep inspiration close by 20
CHAPTER 13   Rest 23
CHAPTER 14   Hire a cleaning service 24
CHAPTER 15   Bathe often 25
CHAPTER 16   Pray 26
CHAPTER 17   Try not to blame your husband 27
CHAPTER 18   Talk with your husband 29

Chapter 19	Encourage your husband to get out for awhile	31
Chapter 20	Don't neglect your teeth	32
Chapter 21	Vent	33
Chapter 22	Keep snacks on hand	34
Chapter 23	Stay Hydrated	35
Chapter 24	Eliminate factors that might be making it worse	36
Chapter 25	Give suggestions a chance	37
Chapter 26	Read testimonies	40
Chapter 27	Don't Miss Out	41
Chapter 28	Treat yourself	42
Chapter 29	Keep a Journal	43
Chapter 30	Acupressure/Acupuncture	45
Chapter 31	Wear loose fitting clothes	47
Chapter 32	Homeopathy	48
Chapter 33	Try different recipes	49
Chapter 34	Have your baby shower at home	51
Chapter 35	Hypnosis	52
Chapter 36	Myofascial Trigger Point Therapy	54
Chapter 37	Request a hospital stay	55
Chapter 38	be sympathetic to others	57
Chapter 39	Seek professional counseling	59
Chapter 40	Prepare for your next pregnancy	62
Chapter 41	Eliminate other possible illnesses	64
Chapter 42	Prenatal Vitamins	65
Chapter 43	Pinch your ear	66

CHAPTER 44	Carry lemon scent with you	67
CHAPTER 45	Massage	68
CHAPTER 46	Eat more beans	69
CHAPTER 47	Steroid Therapy	70
CHAPTER 48	Nutritional therapy	71
CHAPTER 49	Pay it forward	75
CHAPTER 50	Be Thankful	76

Acknowledgements

Above all I would like to thank God for blessing me with a wonderful family.

I would like to express my thanks to my family who helped and supported me through a very difficult time in my life.

I also would like to especially thank my husband Chris for staying by my side and "doing it all" for nine months. He is a great husband and father.

A special thanks to Stefan Boring-Silcott for his computer genius. He was always willing to help when I needed him. Credit goes out to Deanna Dudley for proofreading and giving me feedback to help improve than-you to Mark Sullenbarger for doing the illustrations. My appreciation goes out to April for being such a good friend during it all.

First and foremost, I must express my love for my children Garrett and Grace. They are wonderful blessings in my life and I feel so lucky to be their mommy. They bring me happiness, love, laughter, and peace. And of course they were both worth the wait, or shall I say the agony it took to bring them into this world.

Pregnancy for most women is such a happy time. As it should be you are smothered with attention, women sharing their pregnancy experiences with you. Feeling so material and being so fortunate to be a part of this miraculous process. Shopping for and wearing maternity clothes and the special glow that belongs only to mothers in the making. Picturing all the fun of decorating the baby's room and imagining all the playing and laughter that will take place in it. A time to pick out names for the baby. Wondering what he or she will look like and will the baby resemble Mommy or Daddy.

Now having said that, the first trimester I was pregnant with my son and my entire second pregnancy was the worst experience of my life.

Unfortunately, I might be sugar coating that even a little bit. I suffered with morning sickness every day, all day and night, beginning from week six until delivery. I was actually in the middle of throwing up at the exact moment she was being born.

I have never written a book before, but decided I would give it a try for two reasons. One very selfish reason is to help me put some closure to my horrifying pregnancy experience. It has been three years since my daughter was born and I still find myself trying to resolve issues from that time in my life. I thought it would be somewhat therapeutic if I could write this book of tips and filter in my experience whenever I could. This is my one last attempt to bring an end to this chapter of my life.

The other reason I felt compelled to write this book was to help the other mothers who are going through what I did. I learned from doing research for this book that there were others who experienced cases of HG much worse than mine. It is so unfortunate that in so many mother-to-be books there is only a page or two dedicated to morning sickness and not much more than a definition regarding HG. Women going through this traumatic experience which affects their physical, emotional and mental well being, needs to know they are not alone. Their fear, guilt and frustration are shared among most if not all HG sufferers. It took my whole pregnancy and some time after that to realize things I could have done to make it a little bit easier. I want others to learn quickly what it took me nine months and then some to figure out. I want them to know there are resources out there for when they are in need.

I strived for this book to come across to the reader as a friend with advice who has been in a situation somewhat similar to yours. During my first pregnancy, I read books that's purpose was to educate and help prepare expecting mothers about pregnancy, childbirth and motherhood. Yet, I feel I learned most by the conversations with close friends and family. Their knowledge, special tips, and advice were priceless to me. I simply wanted to have a chance to talk with my HG sisters and share with them all that I have learned.

Lastly, I wanted to make clear that I am not a doctor or "expert" but an HG survivor who learned the hard way on how to cope with being sick

24/7 and all the turmoil it brings. I hope that this book of tips will bring you some hope and relief I know you so desperately need.

Before I get started I thought I would include a definition of Hyperemesis Gravidarum. If you're reading this you more than likely know first hand what it is and you would probably agree that the definition could be summed up best with one word—***HELL!***

Doctors and others may choose to define HG as a condition that includes severe nausea, vomiting, weight loss and electrolyte disturbance. It can lead to dehydration, malnutrition, weight loss, muscle wasting, and emotional turmoil. It can cause a huge strain on marriages, families, friendships, jobs, and finances. It can be so vicious as to bring women to abort due to the severity of the condition.

The reason to why some of us have this and other don't isn't completely understood. Some say hormone levels cause it, multiple pregnancies, and women with weight problems. I have even heard of bizarre causes such as an unwanted pregnancy, TMJ, and a history of wearing braces. We must also be aware that with every pregnancy there is a pretty good chance we will have HG again and more likely worse than before. This is why HG robs many of us who wanted more babies but couldn't face another fight with HG.

1

Call the Doctor's Office Before you Go

Sitting in a doctor's waiting room for a long period of time is excruciating, even when you aren't sick! Nothing gripes me more than being expected to sit in those skinny-ass waiting room chairs forever, just to get called back to another room and wait there sometimes half naked on top of a table, for another long period of time. Ask your doctor if you may call ahead of time and find out if they're running on schedule. If not, have the receptionist tell you when you should arrive to eliminate the wait. The doctor should allow this special exception to help accommodate your situation.

2

Bring someone with you to the appointment

It's helpful to bring someone with you for several reasons. First, your husband, family member, or friend can drive you there and keep you company in the waiting room. More importantly, your companion will be a second set of ears as you talk to the doctor. I don't know how many times I've come home from an appointment and can't remember half of what the doctor said. Have your friend listen closely, and then write down your doctor's comments and suggestions. As you talk with the doctor and tell him how you've been since your last appointment, your loved one can validate what you say and what you've been experiencing. Sometimes the person you bring might even be able to add details. I remember saying as little as possible for fear I'd start crying and not be able to compose myself. Other times, I wouldn't say anything because I wanted to get out of there as soon as possible for fear of getting sick in the office. This person can be your voice. They may be noticing more than you even realize—such as how the nausea and vomiting effects your emotional and mental health while you're focused on your physical health.

This may also help educate your loved one regarding your situation and what you are going through. They may have questions about your condition and what they can be doing for you. Remember, this person, along with other friends and family, may feel helpless and might jump at the chance to come and be there for you.

3

Change your doctor if needed.

You know how sick you are; don't let the doctor tell you otherwise. If your doctor isn't getting it, then spell things out for him. Make him listen. Standing up for yourself right now will be difficult, but it's something you *must* do. I came home from many appointments totally upset with myself for not telling him things he needed to know or asking all my questions. I'd wonder what was wrong with me. Why didn't I speak up? My family would call as soon as I got home wanting to know what the doctor said. They'd ask if I told him how I'd been feeling for the last month. I simply couldn't explain why I didn't ask everything I planned to or why I didn't describe my misery in detail like I promised them I would.

There were times I thought the doctor was so busy I didn't want to keep him any longer than I had to. Maybe I didn't think he could do anything about my problems, especially toward the last trimester, so I thought: Why waste his time? On other occasions, after I thought I'd expressed just how bad I felt, the doctor would say, "Believe it or not a lot of pregnant women feel worse than you do." After hearing this I just felt like giving up. I couldn't imagine feeling worse then I already did. I realize he was right, but it seemed to make me feel as though I didn't even deserve the right to complain or ask for any relief.

Looking back on it now, I realize I didn't have the strength to stand up for myself. I was weak and defenseless. The sickness had taken the energy I needed to be my own advocate.

It's so important that your doctor truly knows what you're going through. Write down what you can—even if it's a small, one word reminder. Give the list to him and discuss it with him. He has to know everything that's going on before he can help you.

If you don't feel you're getting the attention you need from your doctor, then consider a second opinion. An empathetic doctor is essential. You must be able to confide in him or her and feel comfortable and safe doing so. He should be understanding and encouraging you *right now*.

If you do make the decision to change doctors, call your local hospital's OB department and ask for a referral to a physician who has experience with patients who have had HG. Finding a caring doctor who has experience treating HG will help you receive the best treatment possible and might make a huge difference in the outcome of your pregnancy.

4

Lose the guilt.

Guilt can sometimes feel worse than the nausea. You will smother yourself with guilt over things you can no longer control. You might feel guilty because you're taking time off work and therefore not bringing in the income you desperately need. Or perhaps you feel guilt about being unable to take care of your family. I remember saying to myself, "Okay I don't have cancer or some terminal illness. I'm healthy, and there's an end to this in the future. I got pregnant the first time we tried and I'm carrying a healthy baby, so I have no right to complain."

Then there's the guilt of secretly wishing you weren't pregnant, or the thought of not being totally devastated if a miscarriage would happen. Maybe you've even considered abortion. I was guilty of all of these.

I felt like such a terrible mother to my son Garrett, who was approximately eighteen months old when I got pregnant. He was at an age where he needed my attention. His brain was like a sponge and he was eager to learn anything and everything he could. I couldn't be there for him and it was devastating to me. I desperately wanted to play and interact with him, something he would beg me to do daily. But I could barely muster the strength to get his lunch on the days I didn't have any help. I couldn't stop thinking about how I'd never get this time back with him. I was missing out on so much and it broke my heart.

Looking back, I now realize my health problems gave my husband and son more time together, and I think they're closer today because of it. I'm proud and relieved to know my husband is a wonderful father. This experience showed me he's responsible and can take care of my children if anything ever happens to me. My son also became closer to his grandparents and other family members who helped take care of him.

My mother reassured me time and time again, telling me this time was good for Garrett to learn to be more independent. She was right. He needed to learn to play by himself and he did—which helped prepare him to share my attention when his little sister came home.

Remember your situation. You're probably lying down every chance you get—and what else do you have to do but lie there and think? Don't let guilt overwhelm you. You don't deserve this. Let the negative thoughts come and go and recognize they are only thoughts. Talk with your loved ones and let them give you the reassurance you need. Remember, you're doing the best you can given the cards you were dealt. If feelings of guilt begin to consume you, talk to your doctor as soon as possible. He can give you the reassurance you need and treat you effectively.

5

Request time off work if necessary

If you feel like you can't work due to your sickness, call your physician immediately and request a written note to your employer stating you need time off until you're feeling better. Your job should not be in jeopardy if your doctor sends a written statement documenting his orders for you to take off work. You can assure them you'll return as soon as you possibly can. Don't be "quilted" into staying any longer or coming back before you're ready. You will be no help to them if you're sick.

6

Carry trash bag at all times

Buy some unscented two-gallon bags and take them everywhere you go. If you're throwing up, these trash bags are a must. Keep one in the car, in your purse, and beside your bed. When you need to throw up you'll no longer need to bend over a toilet. It's one thing when it is your toilet and you know it's clean, but throwing up in a public toilet is not good. If you're in a restaurant and you feel that urge, go to a bathroom stall, pull out your trash bag, and let her go! It's also convenient in the car if you can't pull over right away. The trash bags even come in handy at home in case someone else is occupying the bathroom and you're desperate. The trash bags are better than a pan or bucket, because no clean up is needed. Another good idea is to carry baby wipes (unscented of course) and a travel size toothbrush and toothpaste in your purse to help you freshen up afterwards.

During my first pregnancy, I went to a community picnic with my husband, his sister and brother-in-law. I'd just entered my second trimester and I was beginning to feel a little bit better. Eager to get out of the house, I jumped at my sister-in-law's invitation to the picnic. I felt fine on the way there, but by the time we arrived I regretted leaving home. I felt absolutely miserable. My sickness came back with a bang! I thought and hoped I might just be hungry (denial), so I ate a hot dog. A few seconds later I was bent over behind a building, not far from where people were mingling; upchucking like it was a sport. I know people had to hear me. I hated to make my husband and his family leave—especially since my husband didn't think it was a good idea for me to go in the first place. But I had to get home! Everyone agreed to go (probably embarrassed to be seen with me), and we got in the van. Without any warning, I had an instant, very strong urge to throw up, which I did, all over myself and the van. There was no time to pull over and I couldn't find anything to throw up into.

So, there I was, throwing up in a Wonder Bread sack my husband found under the seat, while my brother-in-law was reaching from the front seat to wipe puke off my leg. It was mortifying, to say the least.

Please do not subject yourself to this kind of humiliation. Be prepared at all times!

7

Get a haircut

If you have long hair and have always wanted to try a shorter style, now is the time. You really can't lose. Trying to manage long hair can be a nuisance when you're sick. Putting it back in a ponytail is an easy fix and definitely what I suggest if you refuse to cut it. But even if you can put it back everyday, you still have the hassle of washing and combing your hair, not to mention the headaches that come from wearing it up all day.

I was so sick of my long hair that one night I insisted that my husband cut it for me—something I don't recommend! But even if you don't like the new haircut, you'll probably be hibernating for the next few weeks/months anyway, so who do you have to impress? Remember, it will grow back!

8
Hire a babysitter

During my second pregnancy I felt good one week. Whether it was coincidence or not, that same week my sister-in-law was able to baby-sit my son during the day while my husband was at work. At the end of the week I thought I just might be getting over the sickness. The last day she watched him, I felt so good I really could have kept him home. I decided to go ahead and let her watch him so I could get one more day of rest. I felt so much better. I was excited to get back to my normal routine and taking care of my family.

It was the night before Thanksgiving, and I began cooking a dish for the next day, when we were scheduled to celebrate Thanksgiving at my aunt's house. I hadn't been out in forever, and I was looking forward to spending the holiday with my family and eating a wonderful Thanksgiving meal. Then all of a sudden I begin feeling nauseated. *I just need to sit down for a minute,* I told myself. Thinking I might be hungry, I got myself something quick to eat. But the nausea continued and I decided I was trying to do too much too soon and I needed to slow down. I decided to go to bed early to get my rest so I would feel good for Thanksgiving.

I woke up the next day feeling sick. We went to my aunt's house and by this time I was devastated. I'd convinced myself I was done with this. I sat down at the table in front of all that wonderful food, and I felt a big lump in my throat. I knew if someone spoke to me or even made eye contact I'd burst into tears. I excused myself from the table and told my husband I was ready to go. I encouraged him to stay, but explained that I needed to get home because I felt so bad. My sickness continued from that day until I delivered my daughter in March.

The point of all this is that I think I felt good that week because I was able to rest while my sister-in-law babysat my son. Being a stay at home mom is one of the hardest jobs there is, and it's nearly impossible job when you're sick. Surviving a long day with your eighteen month old with no help is absolutely exhausting. As soon as my husband came home I'd begin wondering how I'd get through tomorrow when he returned to work. I contemplated sending my son to daycare. We'd never left him with anyone but family and never for much more than a couple of hours at a time and I worried about how he would adjust. I already felt guilty for not being able to take care of him the way I used to. In fact, it seemed my husband had taken on the role of mother. I could barely take care of him during the day, and by evening I was so worn out that my husband was left to do everything when he got home. He fixed supper, fed our son, bathed him, and prepared him for bed.

If you have the financial resources, I strongly recommend child care. If you don't want to send you child to daycare, there's another option: Hire a sitter to come to your home and baby-sit. You might even consider an older teenager who is certified and wants to earn a little extra cash. Hopefully, you might have a teenager in the family, maybe a niece or nephew. This way you can still be with your child/children. You won't have to worry about who will take him, or pick him up, or how he is adjusting. This will provide you with much needed rest and peace of mind. This in return might give you a little more energy in the evenings and will allow you to accomplish a small task or two!

9

Research

Read all you can on severe morning sickness or Hyperemesis Gravidarum. The more you know, the better equipped you will be to tackle this problem head on. The Internet is an excellent source to help educate yourself on the facts and statistics regarding your condition. If you learn something new or find something interesting or helpful, then don't hesitate to share it with your doctor. More than likely he'll be glad you did. You might even be educating him as well, which in turn will help other expecting moms who are going through the same thing.

You will come across several so-called remedies for morning sickness. Perhaps they come from professionals or mothers who have tried it themselves. But I was always careful to check with my doctor before trying anything new. For the most part, he approved all the things I asked about and I would then try them out. Try not to be discouraged if suggestions aren't working. I tried most everything, from sea bands to sucking on lemons. You never know when a suggestion might be your lifesaver!

Most importantly, you will also come across other pregnant women's testimonials regarding their experience with HG. I strongly suggest you read them. Let these forums be your support group. Read as many as you can. It will make you feel so much better knowing you aren't alone.

My best friend told me her mother was severely sick with both her pregnancies and I desperately wanted to talk with her. I called her one day and pretended I wanted to get a hold of her daughter, and then I started asking her questions and she told me about her experience with HG. I told her it was the first time someone else had described exactly what I was going through. She totally understood and everything she said fit my thoughts exactly. I told her I was having a difficult time keeping up with my son and she told me with her first pregnancy there was no way she could've taken care of a baby. She told me I would never forget how I felt—and she was right. Not a day goes by that I don't think about those times.

10

Ask for help

I believe this is the most important tip of all, and possibly the hardest to follow. Let your family and friends help you. If no one is volunteering, then ask for help. Swallow your pride and guilt and let them lend a hand. It will be healing for them as well. Remember, they're feeling helpless and need to contribute in some way.

I absolutely despised asking for help of any kind. Friends and family would offer and there were times I'd turn them down, thinking I didn't want to put anybody out. I thought they really didn't want to help me and were just trying to be nice.

Taking care of my eighteen month old son was my biggest and hardest responsibility. Caring for him during the day was exhausting and it was a struggle to get through each hour. This is where I needed help the most. Unfortunately, most of all my family members worked full time and weren't available. My father, however, was laid off from work at the time and would come over for a couple of hours each day and watch over Garrett and give me a chance to lie down. I often felt like I was imposing on Dad and would send him home. My best friend would call almost every night and offer to come over and help, but I refused to let her because I knew she had so much on her plate at the time and I didn't want to be a bother to her.

Don't make the same mistakes I made. Let people show their support. Look at it this way: Let them take care of you and make a promise to yourself that you'll be there for them if ever they need you. And you will, because you'll know what it's like to need someone. You will have plenty of chances to return the favors, if not to them, then to someone else in need. Help someone in honor of the person who helped you.

If you have older children in the home, then let them pitch in and help. It will be a good experience and they'll be proud of themselves for what they contribute. This is a good time to add some responsibilities and to allow them to become more independent.

If you don't have family and friends who can help you, then consider resources in your community. Do you belong to a church? Ask your minister or priest for assistance. If you don't belong to a church family, a church may still be willing to help out. Check with your local pregnancy help center, pro-life programs, family health services, or Planned Parenthood. Be sure to present your dilemma to your doctor; perhaps he or she can help you network the area and come up with some assistance. Several web sites regarding HG provide 800 numbers that might be of assistance to you. Call them when you need some verbal support between doctor's appointments; they can give you suggestions on how to cope and manage.

11

Ignore others who doubt you're sick

To this day I wonder if I wasn't sick during my pregnancies because of a judgment I made about a co-worker who was pregnant and battling morning sickness. She changed her work schedule around so she could be off in the morning because of how bad she felt. I remember thinking, *Oh, it can't be that bad—it's just morning sickness.* Well, needless to say, that came around and bit me on the butt! I should have known better then to judge someone like that. Believe me; I paid a price for that mean assessment.

At least I kept the comment to myself, which is better than some of the people who had the nerve to verbally doubt my sickness right to my face. What hurts the most is when it comes from close family and friends.

In the beginning of my pregnancy, I tried using the sea band to help relieve the nausea. I borrowed it from my sister-in-law, who tried it and found it worked for her. I was excited to try it out. I put it on immediately and was told it might take a half hour to forty-five minutes to begin working. It was a weird feeling; it almost felt as though I was getting shocked. Believe me when I say I would have endured this aggravation with a smile on my face for nine months if it worked, but it didn't. I wore the sea band for two straight days and didn't feel one iota better. One day I called and asked a friend to come over and baby-sit Garrett while I lay down for a while. He comes over, saw the sea band on the table, and asked why I wasn't wearing it. I explained that I had tried it for two days and it didn't work. He said I should give it longer to work. If it was going to work I thought it should have already started. I wasn't giving up on it altogether, but was taking a break from the shocking sensations it gave me. I felt he was insinuating I didn't want to get better. Let me just say (and sisters, I know you'll back me up on this) no one would purposely experience nausea every second of every day if they didn't have to. It hurt my feelings to realize that people were judging me.

In their defense, I guess you just don't know exactly what someone is going through unless you've walked in their shoes. Plus, if you love and care about someone, you want desperately to doubt they're suffering so much. However, it doesn't excuse insensitive and tactless remarks. If the people who are passing judgment are just acquaintances or people off the street, then I say don't waste your energy trying to prove otherwise. Let them think what they wish and keep your distance. You deserve support right now, not upsetting accusations.

If the person throwing out disbelief is a close loved one, then try to educate them on the subject of Hyperemesis Gravidarum (HG). Provide them with literature and some written testimonies from different web sites on the Internet that support your description of what you're experiencing. Invite them to join you at your next doctor's visit. Let the doctor convince them that you're sincerely sick. Your loved one can ask questions and become more familiar with what you're going through.

Some time after my HG experience was over my mother got really nauseous after starting a new medication, nausea being one of the side effects, and she remained nauseated for almost two days. She was almost in tears as she apologized to me, explaining she hadn't realized what I had gone through. She said she felt like she could go crazy after two days of nausea and couldn't fathom feeling that way for months without a break. She commented on how she wished she had helped me more than she did after feeling a touch of what I went through. Although I hated seeing her miserable, it was so satisfying to hear those words. Now someone sincerely understands. It is so gratifying when someone gets you, or can truly empathize with total understanding from genuine experience.

If I heard of someone having a terrible hangover I was almost glad so I could say: "You know, that's exactly what I'm feeling every single day, all day and all night long." If I thought they second guessed me in any way, I wanted to lecture them until I felt they believed me.

Again, I say to you: Getting frustrated will only weaken you more. Educate them and include them in everything you learn. Stay clear from those who show disbelief.

12

Keep inspiration close by

When others find out you aren't feeling well, you may start receiving cards from those who want to let you know they're thinking of you. I was fortunate enough to receive a few of these during my pregnancy. I never knew how comforting it is to get these well wishes from friends and family. They are wonderful to receive and can be very therapeutic. Keep the letters open and by your bed side. You will be amazed at how many times you look over and read those cards and messages. They'll remind you to stay hopeful, be patient, and—most of all—that people care about you.

My sister sent me a card in the mail and wrote, "Take one day at a time." I stared at that message over and over, and I soon began thinking more that way. If I could just make it through today, then I would worry about tomorrow later. I realized I was dwelling too much on how many months I had left until I was due. Then I'd stress about how I was going to survive the next four months. I stopped doing that to myself. If I found myself thinking about the duration of the pregnancy, I'd stop and remind myself, "I only need to worry about surviving today."

Another source of inspiration and education is watching Oprah! This program will educate you and give you insight regarding your well-being. It also might help remind you that other people are in worst shape than you right now. If you pay attention and listen to the message, you'll almost always learn something about yourself and find ways to improve your life. Tuning in for one hour a day might help you give you the motivation to tackle the remainder of your sickness.

Here are some quotes that might lift your spirits for today-

"Reading Inspirational and Motivational Quotes daily are like taking my vitamins."—Rosie Cash

"If you're going through hell, keep going."—Sir Winston Churchill

"You have to accept whatever comes, and the only important thing is that you meet it with courage and with the best that you have to give."—Eleanor Roosevelt

"It is not a weakness, but a courageous thing to ask for help. A coward wallows in his own sorrow."—Linda Castor

"No matter how difficult the challenge, when we spread our wings of faith and allow the winds of God's spirit to lift us, no obstacle is too great to overcome."—Roy Lessin

"Heaven knows we need never be afraid of our tears, for they are the rain upon the blinding dust of earth, overlying our hard hearts."—Charles Dickens

"We shall draw from the heart of suffering itself, the means of inspiration and survival."—Winston Churchill

"If we had no winter, the spring would not be so pleasant; if we did not sometimes taste of adversity, prosperity would not be so welcome."—Anne Bradstreet

"There is nothing in life so difficult that it cannot be overcome. This faith can move mountains. It can change people. It can change the world. You can survive all the great storms in your life."—Dr. Norman Vincent Peale

"It isn't for the moment you are struck that you need courage, but for the long uphill climb back to sanity and faith and security."—Anne Morrow Lindbergh

"There are as many nights as days, and the one is just as long as the other in the year's course. Even a happy life cannot be without a measure of darkness, and the word 'happy' would lose its meaning if it were not balanced by sadness."—Carl Jung

:Patience and perseverance have a magical effect before which difficulties disappear and obstacles vanish."—John Quincy Adams"

"Prayer is asking for rain. Faith is carrying the umbrella."—unknown

"When you have nothing left but God, then for the first time you become aware God is enough."—unknown

"Feed your faith and your doubts will starve to death."—Unknown

"God will never lead you where his grace cannot keep you."—unknown

"There will be ups and there will be downs, there will be times when things make sense, and there will be times when they don't, but you'll always be on an adventure of meaning if you live for self, family, and others."—Christopher Reeve

"Please Lord, teach us to laugh again, but God, don't let us forget that we cried."—unknown

13

Rest

This is a huge tip. Never underestimate the need for rest. Not getting the rest you need can worsen the nausea. If you feel like lying down, then do so. Don't try and be super mom or super wife right now. This is a time to take care of yourself and the baby growing inside of you.

There was one week when I felt okay during my pregnancy—the week I mentioned earlier when my sister-in-law helped out by babysitting my son. I was able to rest the entire day, every day. By the end of the week, I truly believed the worst was over.

Then I started trying to pick up where I'd left off when I first began feeling sick. I began doing some cleaning and caught up on the laundry—just getting the house back into shape. I told myself, "I am totally ready for the rest of these nine months. Bring it on!" I was actually looking forward to the next week when I'd be taking care of Garrett without help from anyone.

Then the sickness came back on Thanksgiving Day. I truly think if I would have continued feeling at least a little better if I would've continued to rest and slowly returned to my routine. I came to the conclusion I'd done too much too soon. Unfortunately, I reached this conclusion after my daughter was born (a little late!)

If you don't trust this tip, then I suggest you experiment with a little trial and error. Try it my way one week, and then try it your way the next. Determine which week you felt better!

14

Hire a cleaning service

If you have the financial resources don't think twice about this. Just do it! This is one less responsibility you'll have to worry about. You can usually find cleaning services in your local yellow pages. Having a clean house always made me feel better and I strongly recommend it.

If you are able to afford it you can also have your clothes laundered at a reasonable price. Call around your local laundry mats for some price quotes.

15

Bathe often

This seems like the biggest chore when you're feeling so weak, and it's also the biggest relief when you're finished. I suggest taking baths rather than showers if possible, so you can sit in the tub and relax.

So many times I attempted to take a shower and thought I would die before I was done. I'd be slumped over and in tears by the time I stepped out. Taking a break on the toilet was a must before I attempted the feat of drying off. Then I needed another break before dressing myself, and yet another break before combing my hair. That's why I recommend bathing rather than showering. You can get in the warm water and try to relax for a few minutes. Then when you feel like you need to take a break, you can do so.

Taking your bath at night is often a good idea. Think of it as the last chore of the day. When you're sick with the flu, pregnant, or not feeling well for whatever reason, a bath will help you relax before going to bed.

16

Pray

Have a little talk with Jesus. Trust me when I say you will find yourself in the kneeling position plenty of times anyway. Now, you might be grasping a toilet rather than clasping your hands together, but that's ok. When you're by yourself and need to talk—then talk with Him. It will help you find a little serenity and comfort. Remember, He's always with you!

There were many times I held onto the thought: "He will never give us anything we can't handle." I would ask him for forgiveness for the many complaints I made each day regarding the precious blessing he'd given me. I apologized for not being more thankful for the blessings in my life and for carrying a healthy baby. I would pray out loud, and by the end of my prayer I always felt a little more peaceful.

If you can't attend your church, then consider the following: Read your bible, even if you can only manage a few words at a time. Call a member of your congregation and ask what the sermon was about. Ask your church if the sermon could be audio taped or recorded on video for you. Listen to your favorite gospel music.

17

Try not to blame your husband

This is going to be tough, especially when you rise from a throwing up session and notice he's shoveling a handful of Doritos into his mouth, looking untouched by the misery you're smothered in. You might want to cuss me here, but hear me out when I say to be easy on him—especially if he's trying his best. Believe it or not, this is very hard on him also. It's hard on anyone to see a loved one so sick all the time. This was supposed to be a wonderful time for you both; possibly even an opportunity to grow closer as you anticipated the birth of your baby. I'm sure neither of you seen this curve ball coming.

I have a wonderful husband who did his very best when I was sick. He cooked, cleaned, and took care of our son when he wasn't at work. He took on the role of a single parent. Knowing this, I would still get angry and defensive if he complained about doing both our shares of the workload, or if I heard someone else comment on how great he was to me or say, "Poor Chris, he's really running himself ragged." Excuse me? I would tell him and them I'd gladly trade places with him in a minute! I think I would snap back at him because I hated the fact that he had to do everything and I was feeling so guilty about it. Also, I sometimes resented the fact that he felt fine and looked great when I looked horrid and felt deathly sick. That's why I don't like the expression, "We're pregnant." Let us get one thing straight right now: The mother is pregnant; the father is not!

Despite his complaining, which didn't happen very often, my husband was very patient and for the most part understanding. Now having said this, there were still times when I lost my temper with him. He would comment on how I'd feel better if I got up and started doing something. Or he'd say a lot of the problem was in my head. He also refused to take vacation time to stay home and help me, because he wanted to take off when I had the baby. I would beg him to take his vacation so he could be at home and help me with Garrett. He insisted that I'd need him more when the baby was born. We argued many times over this. He backed up his argument with his sister's offer to baby-sit while he was at work. She already had a toddler and a newborn at home and I thought that would be too overwhelming for her. Plus he wanted me to take Garrett out to her house—which was a huge chore in itself. Besides, I didn't really want Garrett away from me that long. Why did we have to inconvenience her when he could take vacation time? Neither of us would budge.

We were both stressed and put to the test. We were both tired. At times I just had to vent and I took out my frustration on him. This would hurt him, because he thought he was doing his best and not getting any appreciation for it. It definitely took a toll on our marriage—but we did survive it and I think we're now closer. I know now that he's with me for the long run. He definitely proved that he loved and cared about me and our family. We know now we can pretty much handle anything that comes our way. We are definitely stronger because of this (although he still should have taken his vacation!—I guess I'm still not over that one!)

Learn from my mistakes and appreciate your husband. Tell him that you do notice all he's doing and that you are grateful that he's trying. Remember this is hard on you both, so try your best not to place blame.

18

Talk with your husband

Most likely this is new to both of you, so good communication is critical from beginning to end. Often we women think our spouse should know what we're thinking and we get upset if they disappoint us by being clueless. This is not the time to expect him to know anything or to do anything without you telling or asking him. Neither of you know what the other is going through. So tell each other. Never assume he knows. Tell him how you're feeling physically, emotionally, and mentally. Don't assume he knows by the way you look when you're bent over the commode and in tears begging for mercy. You must take time to tell him. If he happens to ask what he can do for you, you must tell him. Don't say, "Nothing, honey," while thinking, *why doesn't he get up, go to the kitchen and put the dishes that have been in the sink for two days, into the dishwasher.* Then when he doesn't do this, but instead plops down in the recliner and turns on football, you get angry. This isn't fair to him. He offered to do whatever you asked of him. It's not his fault you didn't take him up on his offer. I know its difficult to ask things of him when he's tired from working all day, but if he makes an effort to step up to the plate, then give him that chance to help you.

Take time every evening to talk to one another about the day. Tell him what you did and how you felt. Give him a chance to vent about his day as well. Then be sure to let him know you've noticed how hard he's trying. If you don't think he's doing his part, confront him. Try to be supportive. Don't be judgmental over his explanation. Hopefully he'll think about it for a while and come to the conclusion that he can handle more. If he truly believes he's doing his best, then maybe he can arrange for a third party to come in and help. Suggest he might come to your next doctor's appointment and discuss things with your physician.

19

Encourage your husband to get out for awhile

Eventually, your husband will need some time on his own. Encourage him to get out of the house and just get away for a couple of hours. It will do him good to get some much needed time to himself. Perhaps he could get out with friends and do some venting. It will help you as well, because he'll be less frustrated with the situation at home. Hopefully he'll come home in a better mood, again ready to give one hundred percent to the family. Being around a sick person all the time can be frustrating and draining—not to mention a bit depressing (sorry, I had to say it.) Acknowledge this and give him the space and time he needs to refuel his energy and spirit!

20

Don't neglect your teeth

It's important to take extra care of your teeth right now. If you're vomiting often, stomach acid can cling to your teeth and eat away the enamel. Right before brushing try and relax your face muscles. Try using mint toothpaste to freshen your mouth. The mint might also help minimize the nausea. If you find that your tooth paste tends to gag you try switching to kids toothpaste where the taste isn't as strong. Colgate seems not to bubble up so much. Try using a smaller toothbrush or a toothbrush designed for children. Be sure to schedule a dental appointment as quickly as possible after you have your baby to make sure your teeth are free from cavities and are in good health.

21

Vent

Sometimes you just feel better when you let it all out. Get a box of tissues, make yourself comfortable, and have you your own little pity party. Cry your eyes out, sob out loud! Now, when you're all done, pull yourself together, take a deep breath, and tell yourself that you can do this and that you are strong and ready to fight. Declare war on your HG! Be brave and challenge it: BRING IT ON! Yeah! That's right, we said it! We're on like Donkey Kong!

I seemed to cry at least once a day when I was pregnant and sick; it usually happened in the evening. Along about seven o'clock every night I'd have a little crying jag, but I felt better afterwards. It would somehow give me a sense of starting anew. That's when I would tell myself: Take one day at a time. Tomorrow may be better. I can do this.

Holding your emotions in will take a toll on you, so don't be afraid to use crying as an outlet. Give yourself permission to shed some tears; wail if you need to. Shout, holler profanities, growl—whatever makes you feel better. May I suggest you warn whoever is in the house that you're about to blow off a little steam, otherwise they might think you've gone off the deep end! Better yet, wait 'till you're alone in the house!

22

Keep snacks on hand

Keep snacks with you at all times. Carry a little baggie or container with you wherever you go! I suggest peanut butter crackers, saltine crackers, pretzels, lemon drops, peppermint candy, or whatever else you're able to keep down.

23

Stay Hydrated

I know this is easier said than done, but you must drink plenty of fluids—whatever works—because you need to stay hydrated. Try lemonade, ginger ale, or ginger tea. Some have claimed relief by sipping coffee. Be careful of the caffeine, which can sometimes worsen nausea and has also been known to worsen acid reflux. You will find through trial and error what drinks you like best, what works to ease the nausea, and what will stay down. Go with what works. Try and sip slowly to help keep it down. Also try to drink really cold drinks or really hot drinks. The temperature of the drink can also make a difference.

Toward the middle of my pregnancy I wasn't throwing up nearly as much, but the nausea was still strong. The vomiting had decreased, so, I didn't worry so much about getting dehydrated. I continued drinking a lot of water, but I still ended up in the hospital with dehydration.

If you're constantly concerned about whether or not you are dehydrated, purchase a container of Keotostix at the drug store. These are paper sticks you place in your urine to detect dehydration. This will be a wise purchase if it helps to keep you from worrying.

Remember to keep water with you at all times. If you go somewhere, take bottled water with you. At night, keep a glass of water by your bedside. Try eating soup as a snack between meals. When showering keep your mouth open—just kidding!

24

Eliminate factors that might be making it worse

Stress is a huge factor that can trigger nausea. Try and keep your environment as stress-free as possible. If you need to rest, common sense tells you not to lie down in the noisiest room of the house. Go to a room where you can lie down with some peace. Turn the television off and get rid of anything else that might be irritating.

I absolutely love watching television, but when I was sick, the TV got on my nerves. I would have to turn it off and at times swear I wouldn't watch one minute of TV after I had my baby. It usually helps to eliminate noise. If you're going somewhere in an automobile, ask to sit up front to protect yourself from getting car sick. Others should be more than willing to give up shotgun to make the ride more comfortable for you!

If odors bother you, then stay out of the kitchen. Let your husband cook. Grill out if weather permits. If you must cook, then try using the microwave to help eliminate lingering smells in the kitchen. Raise the kitchen window if possible. Politely ask those who are planning a long visit to refrain from wearing perfumes and strong scents. If you don't feel comfortable doing this, then ask your husband or someone real close to you to send the message. Consider changing your soap, toothpaste, deodorant, and whatever else might be triggering you to get sick.

25

Give suggestions a chance

I have to say that I tried almost every remedy suggested to me, after first running it by my doctor. I strongly suggest asking your physician first. I will list for you the remedies that were passed on to me, along with some I've recently learned about:

- Relief Band
- Sea bands
- Bio Band
- Ginger Candy
- Ginger Tea
- Ginger ale
- Pretzels
- Sucking on lemons
- Eating tart and salty foods together
- Cottage cheese
- Eating foods that are high in carbohydrates
- Avoiding greasy foods
- Avoiding spicy foods

- Eat frequently—every two hours
- Avoiding rich foods
- Eating bland foods, such as crackers, noodles, dry toast, potatoes, and rice
- Mix three teaspoons of apple cider vinegar with warm water and drink
- Get out of bed slowly in the morning
- Don't drink with your meals
- Avoid lying down right after eating
- Cook with microwave to help eliminate smells
- Take naps
- Sniff rubbing alcohol

Medications that have been used to help treat hyperemesis gravidarum include, but are not limited to, the following:

Antihistimines

Effective in mild cases. Common side effects include drowsiness, dry mouth, blurred vision, constipation, urinary retention, restlessness, sedation, insomnia, upset stomach, nervousness, and headache. Examples of these drugs include:

- Bonine
- Atarax
- Antivert
- Vistaril
- Marezine

- Tigan
- Dramamine
- Benadryl
- Doxylamine
- Dilectin

Antidopaminergics: Phenothiazines. Common side effects include drowsiness, low blood pressure, dry mouth, constipation, urinary retention, rash, restlessness, confusion, and fatigue. These medications may be helpful in mild and moderate cases and are sometimes used in conjunction with other medications:

- Compazine
- Phenergan
- Thorazine (may increase risk of fetal malformations)
- Haldol

One prescription medicine that seems quite popular with the HG population is Zofran. Unfortunately, I never knew about it while I was pregnant. I have read a lot of success stories from those who have used it. It can be taken in pill form or by a pump delivery system which can be set up in your home via home health aid. It seems to have great results. The only kicker is that it is very expensive. It is definitely worth mentioning to your doctor. What am I saying? It is definitely worth getting on your hands and knees and begging your doctor for a prescription of what some might call a miracle drug!

26

Read testimonies

While doing research for this book I discovered several helpful web sites I only wish I'd knew about when I was pregnant. These sites provide good information that can help you to better understand HG. They are also a great place to read testimonies from real women who've been in your shoes. Reading someone else's story can be extremely healing. You might have feelings of guilt you can't share with anyone, fearing they'll think you're a horrible person. You will be surprised at how many other HG sufferers are feeling the exact same way. You won't believe how similar your experiences are. To this day I still read them, and feel relieved to know I was and am not alone. I read these testimonies and sit there in awe, because they have written exactly what I went through. You will be amazed at how much better you feel emotionally after reading these stories.

These websites also give you a chance to vent your frustration. Tell your story. Ask other mothers what has worked for them and if they have any suggestions for you.

The following websites are wonderful and I highly recommend visiting them as often as you can. You'll be glad you did!

www.sosmorningsickness.com
www.hyperemesis.com
www.morningsicknesshelp.com
www.babycenter.com
www.motherisk.org
www.angelfire.com

27

Don't Miss Out

Just because you're sick and unable to get out don't, miss out on everything. If your children are participating in different activities you can't attend, send a camcorder to capture the event. Ask your husband to take pictures or videotape. If he can't attend, then ask another parent if they'll be willing to tape the event for you. Then, when you get the video, watch it with your children and let them narrate it for you. They'll love the chance to sit and watch the movie with you and see your reaction. This is a good idea for other events as well. Send the camcorder along to weddings, family reunions, birthday parties, etc. This will keep you from feeling left out and give you something to look forward to when the family comes home from a special gathering.

28

Treat yourself

You're sacrificing a lot right now for you and your baby. You should be proud of yourself, but more than likely you're beating yourself up with unjustified feelings of failure and guilt. That's why it's important to treat yourself whenever possible. You absolutely deserve it! At least once a week do something for <u>you</u>. Celebrate lasting through another week! This is a huge accomplishment, so don't downplay it. May I suggest a pedicure? At least you can sit down and rest during the procedure. Or go to a movie. Here too, you can sit down and rest while you watch it. Maybe you'd enjoy a little shopping trip? Before you claim there's no way you could go shopping in the condition you're in, remember the home shopping channel! You can shop while lying on the couch. Pretty convenient huh?

Maybe the best gift would be to cut you a little slack. Don't be so hard on yourself. Realize what you are going through and then take credit for what you've earned. Don't be modest—pat yourself on the back for these weeks or months you've survived.

Treating yourself can help you take a small break from the hell you're going through right now. If something gets your mind off your sickness for even an hour or two it will be so worth it.

29

Keep a Journal

Keeping a daily journal is just another way to get your emotions out. Writing them down on paper is a great way to have a little conversation with yourself. If you don't feel well enough to write, then ask someone to write while you dictate. Another alternative would be to audio record your journal and then write it down when you feel better.

Writing at nighttime will help bring closure to each day—another indicator that you've survived yet another calendar day and are twenty-four hours closer to the finish line!

Keeping your journal to read after the baby is born is a good idea. I believe this is healing and it validates what you actually went through. You won't think back and wonder if it actually was as bad as you remember. You can read a few pages and know your memory is correct. It can sometimes take a while to get over this traumatic experience. When you tell yourself you should be over it by now, go back and read your journal and realize yet again what you went through.

It would be great if you could keep a journal regarding your diet, weight and how often you are vomiting. Be sure to bring your journals with you to your MD appointment to help determine which foods are staying down and which foods to avoid. Your journal just might help you discover what diet works best for you.

The following page is an example of a journal you could use. Make copies of this page to use or simply make your own whichever you prefer!

My Morning Sickness Journal

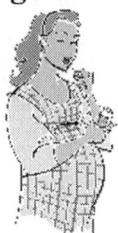

Date/time	Foods	Drinks	Nausea Scale 1-10	Vomiting #times	Weight	Medications	Exercise Yes/No

30

Acupressure/Acupuncture

Alternative therapies such as Acupressure and Acupuncture deserve at least a conversation between you and your doctor. Many mothers would feel it important to consider before drug therapy. There is however contradictions regarding the overall safety of these treatments. Some research claims it is very safe while other studies find these methods could have possible effects to the fetus during early pregnancy and it could also induce labor.

The theory behind these practices is that the body is somewhat experiencing an imbalance which then leads to weakness which can lead to disorders. These practices help bring the body back into balance.

Acupuncture, a traditional Chinese medicine, involves placing needles at certain points on the body. This should be performed by someone who is certified. To find a practitioner contact-

    NCCA
    P.O. Box 97075
    Washington, DC 20090-7075

For a small fee they will send you a list of certified practitioners.

If you fear needles, there is an alternative that offers the same results but is much less invasive. This is called full spectrum light therapy. Instead of using needles, stimulation is made by wavelength light aimed at the same points as acupuncture. The great thing is that it can be administered by YOU. The treatment should last about five minutes. There is no harmful effect if you are off your target. It will however minimize the effectiveness of the results. You can order the kit for approximately $200. For more information you can e-mail SpectrumTherapies@barbeckbb.com or call their too free# (866) 881-0533.

Acupressure, a cousin to the acupuncture, has also been found to bring relief for nausea. This method uses fingers and elbows on certain trigger points. This helps free the flow of energy bringing balance to the body. Relief bands provide this work for you. They can be described as a band that goes around your wrist much like a watch. There is a part on the band that is to be manually placed on the trigger point that brings relief. Some find the relief comes quite quickly while others aren't so lucky. It can be prescribed by your doctor or you can purchase one yourself for a small cost at your local drug store.

It would be a good idea to check with your insurance company to see if they cover any of these services. I hope I haven't put any "pressure" on you to try this remedy (HAHA-get it?-pressure).

31

Wear loose fitting clothes

Try and dress as comfortably as possible. Anything tight around your stomach could aggravate the nausea. Keep it loose! During my pregnancy, I lived in sweat pants and loungewear. Make efforts to stay away from blue jeans at all costs. Throughout the day when you do find a heavenly chance to lie down, blue jeans will not be relaxing. If the weather is warm, I suggest loose fitting shorts. It's imperative that you stay cool, because (you guessed it) heat will worsen your nausea!

Although staying in pajamas is the ultimate solution for some, others might feel guilty doing so—though this guilt is totally not deserved. Some women feel better if they get dressed early on. Whatever your style, I recommend comfort before cute!

When you change clothing, decide whether your clothes need to be washed or can they take one more day of wear? Take into account how much laundry will build up if you carelessly throw everything in the hamper even though you only wore it a short time.

32

Homeopathy

This method has been around for approximately two hundred years. Homeopathic remedies are known to be safe and can be purchased over the counter. Homeopathy is effective in treating the whole person—physically, mentally and emotionally—and all three of these areas are important to the pregnant mother suffering from HG!

If you decide to give homeopathy a try, I strongly advise you to find a licensed homeopath with experience. The earlier you meet with this practitioner, the better. Before conception would be ideal. You will need to meet the homeopath and answer questions that will no doubt leave you wondering why in the world they need to know such things. Remember, they're about the "whole you." Prepare to be there for a couple of hours answering a variety of questions. If you don't feel up to a long appointment, ask if he or she can come to your home. It never hurts to ask! Let them know your situation and they might be able to accommodate you somehow. Perhaps part of the interview could be done over the phone. It also might take some time for the practitioner to narrow your problem down and select a particular remedy. Don't give up if you try what they suggest and it doesn't work. Meet back with them and let them know the results. This is a process, so don't get discouraged. Inform your doctor of your decision to consult a homeopath. He might be able to make a referral. Keep him informed of your progress.

33

Try different recipes

Some women swear by a specific food or recipe that got them through their pregnancy. If someone mentions a food that helped them, then take a chance on it! I've provided a few recipes that have been known to help. Good luck!

Banana—Orange Shake

2 cups orange juice (try to get calcium enriched juice)
2 bananas, peeled and sliced or mashed
1 cup of ice cream
Put all ingredients in a blender. Cover and blend until smooth.

Quick Shake

1 (13oz.) chilled evaporated milk
½ cup of instant cocoa powder
2 cups vanilla ice cream, softened
Put all ingredients in a blender and blend until thick and smooth.

High Protein Milk

1 quart of milk
½ cup powdered milk
Mix, then chill. This milk may be used in cooking. Serve ½ to one cup portions with or between meals. Makes 1 quart of milk

Chocolate Milkshake

¾ cup high protein milk
1 tablespoon instant cocoa mix
1 scoop ice cream, vanilla or chocolate
Blend ingredients with an egg beater or in blender. Makes 1 to 2 servings
VARIATION: Substitute other flavorings and flavors of ice cream

34

Have your baby shower at home

If you aren't feeling up to it, consider postponing the baby shower until after you've had the baby. I do totally understand if this isn't an option. Every mother wants to have things ready and in place when the baby comes. And why should you be cheated out of another fun and exciting part of pregnancy? May I propose this idea: Have the baby shower in your home. This way you can be comfortable on your big day. This idea will probably thrill the person or people who are throwing the shower, because it will help eliminate costs. Besides, you won't have to bother with trying to load all your gifts and get them home. Instead of the boring baby shower games that take up so much time, they can make their time more useful. Maybe everyone can pitch in and take on a project. Some could work together and help assemble a baby swing, stroller, or work on the baby's room while you delegate. If there aren't enough baby preparations to go around, then give them a dust rag and put 'em to work. I bet everyone will have a great time working together; probably sharing stories of how they did their baby's room, or what kind of stroller they had and how it compares to yours.

While you're resting and watching everyone pitch in, take some pictures. After you have the baby, send your guests thank-you notes along with their pictures. For example, if you have a picture of your aunt helping to assemble a stroller, then take another picture of your baby in the stroller and send them both to her. She'll know how much you appreciated what she did!

35

Hypnosis

Some believe in hypnosis and some do not. I know it is difficult right now being judgmental towards anything that might release you from HG. I have said it before and I'll say it again-if it is safe, GIVE IT A CHANCE! Learn what you can about how hypnosis works and what all it entails. Then when you decide it is all a bunch of nonsense, TRY IT ANYWAY! There have been studies showing where hypnosis was very successful in Hyperemesis Gravidarum cases.

Hypnosis is defined best as a focused state of intense concentration. It is known to be very safe. It can be beneficial to your mental state. During Hypnosis, exploring all the factors which might be aggravating your HG, might help you gain, which might be aggravating your HG, might help you to gain a little bit of control over your sickness. It might be able to assist you with tools to help you to ease your tension, and help with relaxation.

Apparently, a healthier mental state is not all that Hypnotherapy seems to offer. It can be used to help minimize your nausea as well. The theory is that we HG sufferers are more vulnerable to our pregnancy hormones and how they are incredibly imbalanced. In our brain there is an area that is in control of this. Much like when our bathroom scales are off five pounds and we have to adjust it back to zero. Hypnosis can help regulate the nausea center in our brain.

Good news is that insurance companies will sometimes pay for the session if it is performed by a counselor that is a certified Hypnotherapist. Consult with your doctor about your interest in hypnotherapy and ask for a referral. You can also contact the American Society of Clinical Hypnosis. They should be able to provide you with a list of qualified hypnotherapists around your area. You may reach them by phone (630 980-4740) or by e-mail at info@asch.net.

While studying up on hypnosis and how it could help eliminate HG, I stumbled across a website providing information about a remedy called "Morning Well." This is a sound remedy that was first used to help stop motion sickness while traveling. A couple of women contacted DAVAL, the company who makes the tape, and asked if it could help morning sickness. They tried the tape and found it indeed helped.

Lynne Mayo, a Community and Birth Center Midwife, handed out the Morning Well tapes to any of her clients who complained of morning sickness. She says the tapes were successful. For some clients the tape stopped the symptoms completely, and for others it eased their symptoms. There were some who didn't experience a difference, but that was a small percentage compared to the number of women who it had helped.

The tapes are said to be totally safe for the mother and the baby and must be used with a personal stereo. They can be ordered off the Internet and cost around twenty dollars. You can read testimonials from women who've tried the Morning Well tape and they are very promising. I wish I'd known about this when I was pregnant!

Speaking of tapes, if you can't afford the Morning Well, or until you receive it, try listening to relaxation tapes. It may not help your sickness, but it might help lessen the tension and calm you down a bit. Try this exercise after one of your venting episodes:

Go to a quiet room where there will be no traffic or interruptions. Put on some comfortable lounging clothes and lie in a relaxing position with your feet out and your palms up. Turn on the relaxation tape, and concentrate on relaxing every inch of your body. You deserve this time to yourself. You may be amazed by the positive impact this will have on you.

36

Myofascial Trigger Point Therapy

This method works by relieving the Pyloric Sphincter spasm that initiates HG. A registered nurse who worked with women with difficult pregnancies found this procedure worked. She performed it on the pregnant mom when she was admitted to the hospital for dehydration from HG. You need someone other than yourself to help perform the procedure, because the pyloric sphincter area is sometimes too tender for the mom to do to herself. The person applies pressure on the area pointed out in the diagram. There's a chance you might feel nauseated right afterwards (what's new?) Be patient, you should get relief in just a bit. You will need to repeat this every three hours. If this area is too tender, then try every six hours.

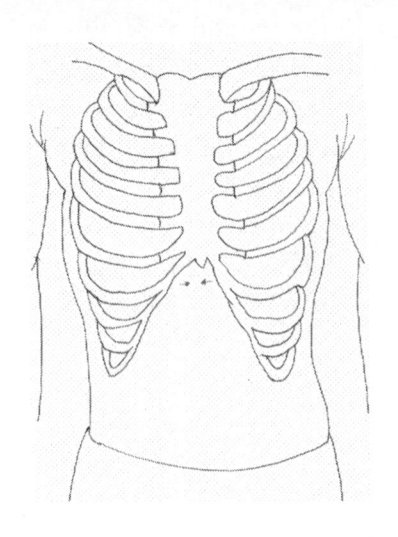

37

Request a hospital stay

If you feel you aren't getting adequate rest or care at home, then talk with your physician about spending a couple of days in the hospital. Talk with your doctor and explain that you desperately need relief. He may totally agree with you, or at least help you come up with a better solution. If what he suggests doesn't work, then bring up the hospital stay again. Check with your insurance company and see what they will cover. Sometimes it's important to contact them immediately before your hospital stay to inform them you're being admitted or they may not cover as much (it happened to me). If this is too much for you to handle, then give your husband or a loved one the information and ask them to contact the insurance company and do the required paperwork.

I was in the hospital one time for two days during my second pregnancy. My family was worried about me and decided to take me to the hospital whether I wanted to go or not. I couldn't put up much of a fight, even if I wanted to! I hoped they would hook me up to an IV for a few hours for re-hydration, and that might help a little. My mother drove me there and did all the talking to the nurse, which was really good because at that point I was in no shape to answer questions. I was physically and emotionally drained. I told myself, *this has to work or I don't know if I can stand anymore.*

The nurse telephoned the doctor and he gave orders to admit me. I'm sure they thought my family would go nuts on them if they didn't do something for me. At that point my family had reached their wits' end.

Come to find out, I was very dehydrated and they hooked me up to an IV right away. I tried to get as comfortable as I possibly could in a hospital bed, with nurses coming in every so often to check my blood pressure and the IV. Even with these disturbances, I was able to rest better than at home. I knew I could let go of all my responsibilities for awhile. All I needed to worry about was getting rest. I remember wishing my visitors would go so I could just lie there and do nothing. My sister brought me a magazine and it was literally too much for me to flip through it and look at the pictures.

The nurses were sympathetic, and it was nice to know they truly believed how bad I felt. One nurse mentioned the woman who was in the next room was also sick, but she was due any day. I was so envious of her because she was at the end of her pregnancy.

During my stay I was able to talk with an OB doctor who was making rounds that day. He came in and sat on my bed and talked with me. He was so gentle and understanding and I felt such an instant trust in him that I revealed my guilt about considering an abortion if I didn't get any better. I wanted to defend my thoughts, so I went on to tell him this was a planned and wanted pregnancy, but I didn't think I could endure anymore sickness. He was sympathetic and said that my feelings were understandable considering what I'd been through. This conversation alone was worth my trip to the hospital.

I left the hospital not feeling any better physically, but much stronger emotionally. I was glad I stayed, because it validated to doubting friends and family members that I actually was sick.

Remember to check with your insurance company for steps to take regarding your hospital admission. My husband had the hardest time getting insurance to cover my stay because they claimed we were suppose to call and notify them (pre-certify) before I was admitted into the hospital.

So keep in mind, if it gets to the point where you can't take it anymore and you feel like you've tried everything under the sun, then tell your doctor immediately and consider a day or two in the hospital to catch up on rest and hydration.

38

be sympathetic to others

Yes, you! I know this is hard to grasp right now, and you probably won't agree or forgive me for saying this, but take it from me: the day will come when you think back to this terrible time and wonder not how others treated you, but how you treated others. You don't need to tell me your excuses about why you aren't your old merry self. I truly understand that from the bottom of my heart. Just know that this isn't easy on the people around you. If you're counting on them to be patient, understanding, and sympathetic, then you must make an effort to do the same.

Not many are going to go out of their way to pitch in and help unless they get a little appreciation. A sister who takes time to do your laundry shouldn't be criticized on how she folds the clothes! Be sure to thank people graciously when they help. A little gratitude goes a long way.

Now I know it's important to vent, but there is a time and place. No one expects you to be Miss Congeniality right now, so if you do have an outburst or say something you wish you hadn't, then be sure to apologize. Even we HG sufferers must take some responsibility for our actions. Apologizing will help you not stress about it and will again remind your victim that you aren't yourself right now.

I hurt someone who is very close to me (and probably others I didn't even know about) by accusing her of not being there for me and helping out more. I thought she could have done more and I held a grudge about it for some time after my daughter was born. I regret that now. Instead of judging her on how much she was helping, I should have been thankful for what she did do. I thought she should have volunteered more without me having to ask her. Now I take responsibility for not asking her for more help. I was too stubborn to ask her, thinking I shouldn't have to. That was my fault.

Again, simply take the time to acknowledge how you're treating the people you love. They care about you, so don't hesitate to tell them you know how much they're doing and you appreciate them.

39

Seek professional counseling

At some point during your pregnancy, you may feel like you're about to lose your mind. You poor thing, you've been hit with a double whammy. You're facing everything that comes with pregnancy—the hormone changes, mood swings, all the high-low emotions—plus you're also dealing with everything that goes along with HG. No wonder you're a basket case!

Another day of this nausea and you swear you'll go insane. You become hopelessly depressed after countless days of feeling so sick. This feeling is almost inevitable. Who wouldn't feel like going nuts after months of severe nausea? The letdown alone after reaching the end of that long first trimester only to find no relief, is enough to make you crazy. Being cooped up in the house lying down all the time, feeling worse than you look, not socializing with the outside world, the constant question of whether this will ever end; these things will bring a good strong woman to her knees.

I was miserably depressed and thought if I could tough it out until after the baby was born I'd be okay. I thought I would be miraculously better the second I delivered. I did feel physically better, but the depression continued. I couldn't understand it. I'd dreamed and begged for this day. I don't know if it was my hormones going wild, or if it was because of the nine months of pure hell I'd just survived. Maybe subconsciously I felt it was finally okay for me to break down (not good timing, considering I now had a toddler and a newborn to take care of). When I found myself crying day and night, I finally went to talk with a counselor. I soon began feeling better and stopped going to my appointments—another mistake. This was a huge ordeal I'd gone through and thinking I should be over it wasn't fair to myself. Even though the pregnancy and sickness ended, along with most of my postpartum depression, I continued to be effected by thoughts of the whole experience everyday. I continued holding grudges against people I loved who didn't offer the support and help I needed. I hadn't yet realized the ordeal that had affected my entire being for nine months wasn't going to go away overnight.

Some time after my daughter was born; my husband and I went along with friends for a much needed night out. During the evening my husband began to get sick and wanted to go home early. Normally, I would have quickly left with him and gone home to help him feel as comfortable as possible. But after nine months of him refusing to stay home and help take care of me and our son, I was out for a little revenge. I told him I'd drive him home and drop him off and then return to the party. I took him home, showing no sympathy, and barely stopped the car long enough for him to get out. Now, I did feel a little guilty about this. The next day he was feeling much better and after some thought and regret I apologized and explained that I wanted him to get a little taste of what I felt like. I shouldn't have done that to him; I know he did his best. But I can't lie—it did feel a little good!

Another red flag that suggested I wasn't quite over my ordeal was the fact that I felt I still needed to tell everybody what I'd gone through, sometimes more than once. My close friends and family bless their hearts; have heard the story a million times. All someone would have to do was mention the word pregnancy, sick, depressed, nausea, babies, morning sickness, and I was off and running—describing what I'd gone through. I pity the person who was foolish enough to mention anything pertaining to the subject.

I think I needed to talk about it and get it out of my system. In fact, that's one reason I decided to write this book: not only to help those who are suffering with the same problems I experienced, but also it was another chance to tell my experience. Besides, I've already talked about it with everyone I know and then some.

Please keep in mind that the effects of HG are not only physical. It's a cancer to our whole being. Yes, it's important to get treatment for the nausea, dehydration, and weight loss, but it's also imperative that we treat the damage caused by the stress of this traumatic experience. Talk with your doctor and consider professional counseling to help bring closure to this chapter in your life and give back to you a healthy body, mind, and spirit.

40

Prepare for your next pregnancy

If you dare to plan another pregnancy after this one, I applaud you! You are one tough woman. It has been said that HG worsens with each pregnancy. This was very true in my case and I've read it's true for other women as well. The good news is, I also know of some women who experienced a much better pregnancy the next time around! Not willing to take that chance my husband was quickly scheduled for a vasectomy after my daughter was born.

Just in case you might be plagued again, then it's best to be prepared. First things first: talk with your boyfriend or husband. Does he want to go through this again? Remember you're not the only one who is affected by HG. Your husband and family might not be too thrilled to see you suffer through another pregnancy. Be sure this is something you both want. Your relationship must be strong and both of you must be prepared to endure what HG might bring the next time around.

If you both decide to try it again, be sure to consider the best timing for you and your family. When can your husband take his vacation? Is there a season during which he works more hours than usual? This pregnancy will be different because now you have a child to consider. Think about who might be available to help. If you contemplate daycare, then obtain the needed information now and determine which one is right for your child. When you're sick is not the time to go inspecting daycare centers. There might also be a waiting list before they can accept your child, so perhaps you can discuss your situation and see what you both agree on.

You may want to consider some dietary changes about a year before you get pregnant. A Harvard study found women with a high intake of saturated fat were more likely to experience severe morning sickness. So cut back on that saturated fat!

Take time to prepare meals and freeze them. Be sure to keep in mind what foods might not go over so well when you're sick. Even if you're unable to eat these meals, your family will benefit from your forethought.

Remember you might be entering nine months of hibernation, so it's not a bad idea to stock up on non-perishable items. Make a list of things you will need that you can purchase now, such as laundry supplies, toilet paper, paper towels, shampoo, soap, cleaning supplies, etc.

Speaking of cleaning supplies now is the time to do your spring cleaning. Get your carpets, windows, and curtains cleaned, because we both know this won't be getting done for some time after the baby is born!

If you really want to get geared up for this next pregnancy then consider doing some early Christmas shopping. You can even go as far as to wrap all your presents and store them away until the holidays. Don't forget about birthdays and other special occasions. If you weren't pleased with the doctor you had during your first pregnancy, then begin your search now. Ask around town or call a referral service to request a recommendation. Make an appointment and talk to the prospective doctor about your last pregnancy and see how she responds. Is she an empathetic doctor? Does she seem eager to provide the best care? Has she/he had previous patients who had suffered from HG, and how did they handle their cases? Ask what you could be doing to help you have a better pregnancy this time around. If this is the doctor you choose, then you should request prenatal vitamins if you haven't already started taking them.

Schedule an appointment for a dental check up. Making sure your teeth are in good condition can help eliminate problems with your teeth during pregnancy. The last thing you need is to be sick and have a toothache to boot!

It's wise to get a flu shot—especially if you're planning a pregnancy that happens to fall during flu season. I recall being pregnant and hesitant about getting a flu shot because I worried it might harm the baby. My doctor actually highly recommended it and provided me with a note regarding his approval.

41

Eliminate other possible illnesses

Sometimes during this wretched pregnancy you'll probably wonder if you might be suffering from something other than HG. Personally, I wanted my sickness to be caused by something else so the doctor might actually be able to do something for me. I recall getting blood work done and being so disappointed when the tests came back normal. The doctor had to remind me it was a good thing that this wasn't related to anything else. I couldn't help but feel differently.

Other ailments your doctor might check for may include but won't be limited to the following;
Gastrointestinal problems
Thyroid problems
Other metabolic disorders
Liver problems
Neurological disorders
Molar pregnancy
Hellp Syndrome

42

Prenatal Vitamins

Having HG and trying to take you prenatal vitamins can be quite a challenge. Some will say their prenatal vitamins make their sickness worse. Some say take your prenatal vitamin in the middle of the day, and others will tell you to take them before going to bed. Some say taking it with your meals work better while others insist on taking their prenatal vitamin after their meal. Talk with your doctor about switching to a different vitamin and see it that seems to help. You can try requesting smaller tablets or possibly capsules that you can break open and pour over your food or in your drink. There are even such things as chewable vitamins that could take care of the problem if swallowing the pill is the problem.

Do not just stop taking your prenatal vitamins without consulting with your doctor first. Your prenatal vitamins contain essential nutrients such as folic acid that will help prevent possible birth defects such as spinal bifida. Through trial and error you and your doctor will work together to find out how you can consume the nutrients you and your baby needs.

43

Pinch your ear

You aren't delusional—you did read this correctly. I know nothing is too bizarre to try and that's the very reason I included this tip. I know the desperation you're in right now and I figure it doesn't cost any money or much energy, so what the heck? Try it and not tell anyone!

It's a simple technique. Place your finger inside your earlobe, at the entrance to the ear canal, and then move your finger to the outer edge of your ear. Some people have a little bump on the outer edge. When you feel this bump you're in the right area. Now squeeze this area for approximately thirty seconds. If you don't feel relief, you can squeeze for up to two minutes. You may also switch ears.

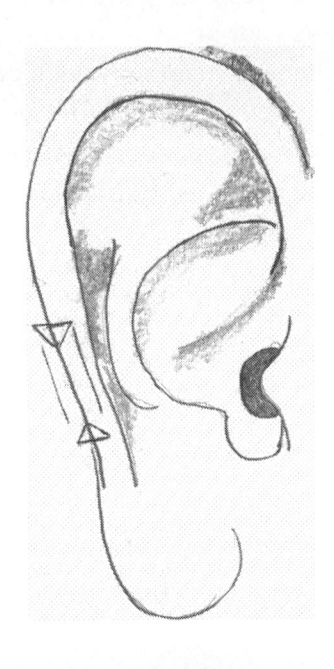

44

Carry lemon scent with you

Lemons are said to be good for easing your nausea. I heard about this during my fifth month and was quick to try it. One day while at a restaurant I ordered lemon with my water. I squirted it into the water and then wrapped up the lemon to suck on during the ride home. I actually think it did help a little bit. I was by no means cured, but for about an hour I didn't hate life, which was a blessing.

Try adding lemon to your diet whenever possible. Drink lemonade, which will be hydrating as well. Suck on lemons or candy lemon drops. Some women have found relief just by smelling lemons. Soak a handkerchief in lemon juice and then let it dry. Fold it up and take it with you for times when you come across a scent that worsens your nausea. Take your handkerchief out and bury your nose in it; hopefully it will alleviate an emergency trip to the bathroom!

45

Massage

Some women find relief from getting a massage especially if you're lying for long periods of time. I personally couldn't stand being touched while I was pregnant and couldn't find any comfort when my husband would offer a back rub. Although I didn't benefit from it, doesn't mean it won't work for you. Be sure to get your doctor's approval and ask if he can make any referrals. Be sure that you go to a massage therapist who's licensed and has had experience with pregnancy massages.

Another option to think about discussing with your doctor is how a chiropractor might help. Some doctors might hold strong negative opinions about chiropractic medicine. Acknowledge their opinion and then request permission to give it try. Ultimately, you should follow your doctor's orders unless you wish to seek a second opinion.

46

Eat more beans

I could write pages explaining the theory of how beans can help, but I'll be kind enough to sum it up for you. Legumes such as pinto beans, kidney beans, garbanzo beans, black eyed peas, lentils, black beans, red beans, navy beans, white beans great northern beans, crowder peas, yellow eyed beans, soup beans, are high in soluble fiber. The soluble fiber in these beans work like a magnet, attracting the bile that builds up in your stomach and causes you to feel sick. The soluble fiber will bind with the bile until it exits through the body. Relief could be found as quickly as after the first serving of beans, but unfortunately it won't last long. When you begin to feel bad again, fix yourself another bowl of beans. Eventually the beans will rid most of the bile and you won't need to consume as much as you did at first. Just remember, beans beans, the more you eat the better you feel, so let's eat beans with every meal!

47

Steroid Therapy

Steroid therapy has proven to win a few battles against HG. Although it does show promise, I would feel much more confident if there were more research that was done to ensure the safety. From what I gathered from my research is that Canada has really embraced it and finds it to be very helpful in many cases. The United States still seems to be skeptical in using steroid therapy to combat HG. Tapering off the steroids almost as quickly as starting them seems to be vital in keeping this therapy safe for the baby.

Of course it shouldn't be the first treatment used in efforts to find relief but when nothing else is working and both the mother and baby's life are in danger it should be at least recognized as a potential solution. It comes down to which harm the baby more—malnutrition from HG or the possible could side effects from the steroids.

48

Nutritional therapy

When you are dehydrated and have lost over 5%of your pre-conception body weight it is time to begin talking about nutritional therapies. Only when all possible options have been attempted, and there is danger of vitamin deficiencies and loss of nutrients should you begin to consider this. Two routes to mull over would include the Picc Line and the Nasogastric Eternal Feeding; both have their pros and cons. Both should only be considered when everything else has failed.

A Picc line is a catheter inserted in your arm by needle and it is threaded into a larger vein located close to the heart. Once it is in position, the needle is removed. The area where the catheter was inserted will be covered with dressing and then taped to your skin. After this procedure has been done you will then have a chest x-ray to make sure the catheter is in the right spot. You can go home with your Picc line in place.

With proper care and support the Picc line can be successful and life saving for you and baby. This is not to say there are not serious risks that must be weighed. Catheter insertions alone may cause life threatening complications. Other possible problems that could result from Picc lines are pancreatitis, Refeeding Syndrome, infections, Septic complications, Hyperglycemia, Hypoglycemia, Essential fatty acid deficiency, electrolyte imbalance, Fluid volume disturbances, and Acid/base imbalance. Talk with your doctor and carefully weigh out the benefits versus the risks.

Nasogastric Enternal Feeding (also known as Nasogastric tube feeding) is an alternative route to obtain nutritional therapy. It involves a small tube inserted in the nose. Nutrients pass through the tube and ends in the stomach. The good news is that it is considered much safer than the PICC line, plus it is cheaper. Women have reported that they do feel less nauseous very quickly after the nasogastric tube is in place. However, I must let you know that I did read a testimony where the woman did not feel much better and did not like the tube inserted in her nose and wanted it out immediately. She was not treated with much compassion. They would not remove the tube at her request and she was forced to keep it in until the next day. Some find it extremely uncomfortable and some find it quite bearable. Weigh out the pros and cons before making your decision. Again these are routes that should only be considered if all other efforts have failed.

Tabby L. Silcott 73

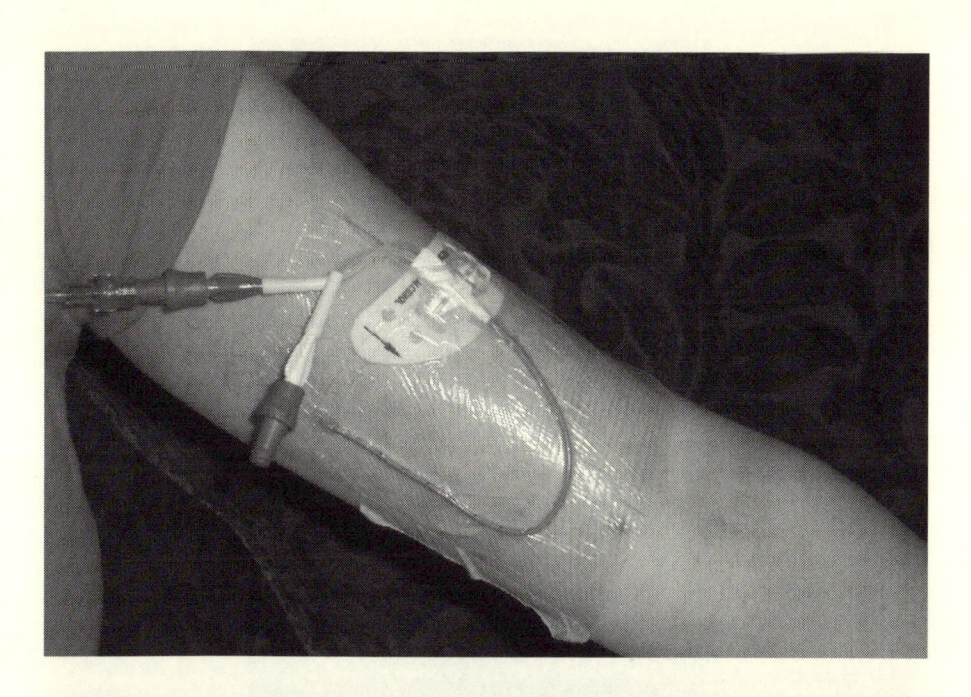

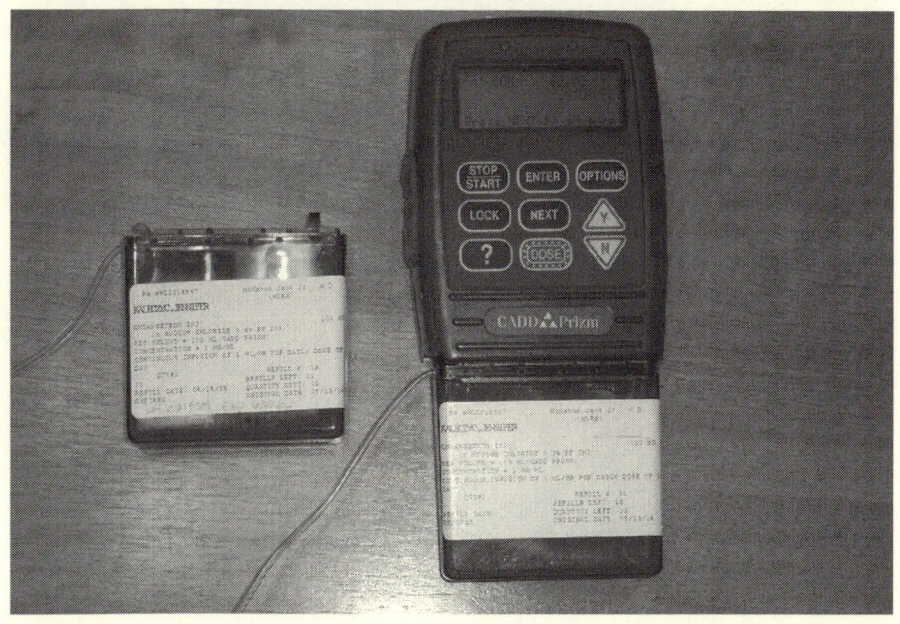

74   Morning Sickness 24/7

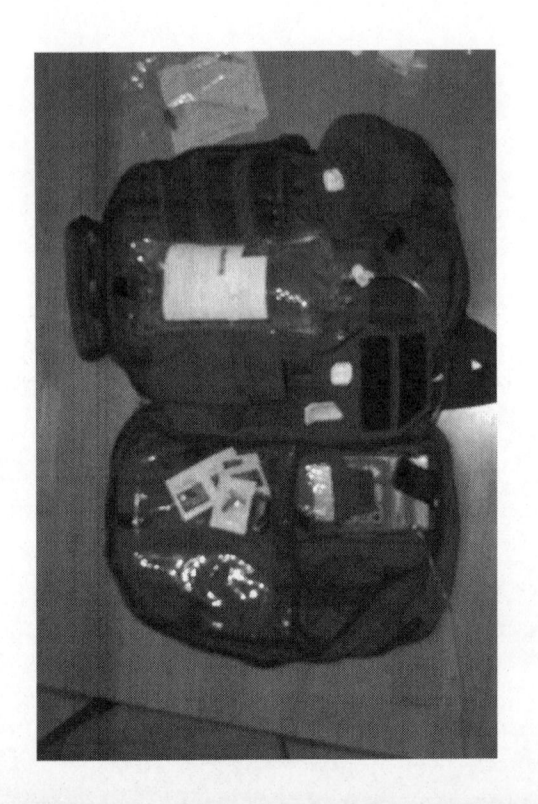

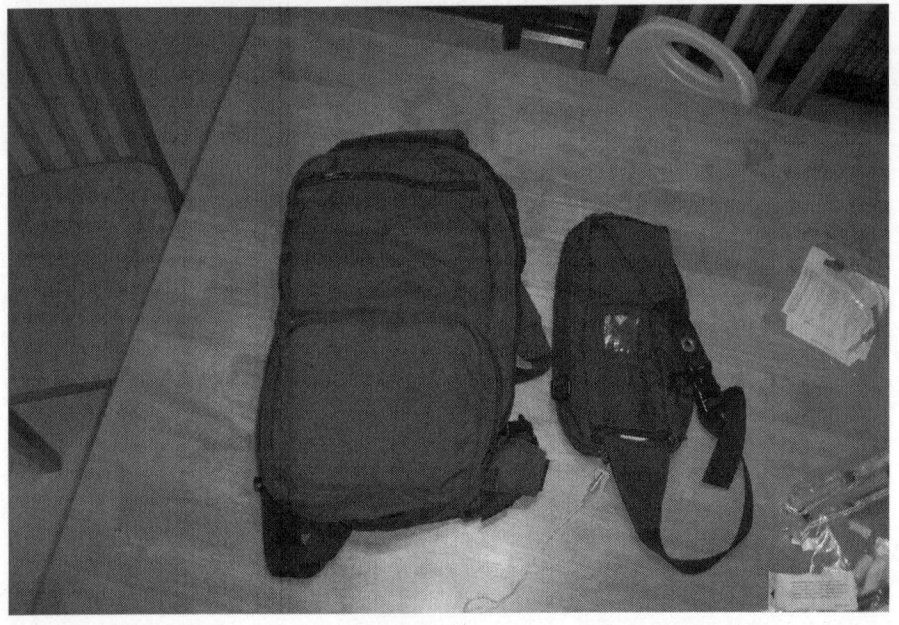

49

Pay it forward

Many times during your pregnancy you'll ask the question "Why me?" Especially when you go out (on those rare occasions) and see other pregnant women who have that special glow and look as though they're happy and enjoying every minute. You can't help but feel cheated.

I struggled with "Why me?" during my entire pregnancy. To this day I still don't have an answer. I did come to the conclusion I wasn't going to go through it for nothing.

I truly feel that we HG sufferers are obligated to help out other pregnant women who struggle as we did. We need to stand together and make a difference. I sure wish I had a mentor during my pregnancy.

Promise yourself now that you will help a HG rookie in the future. Whether it's someone in your own town who can use a homemade dinner and encouraging words, or someone on one of the websites I mentioned earlier—you can make a difference. Volunteer at one of the websites to support a mother in need. You can communicate with that mother via e-mail or by letter or telephone, whatever you are most comfortable with. Monetary donations are needed by different foundations trying to spread education and support for finding relief for HG victims. We can't let what happened to us be all in vain. We are strong women who can help empower others! Remember that helping this cause will in turn help you have closure regarding your own HG battle!

50

Be Thankful

Yeah, you read it right. It's a good thing I'm writing this because I never would have the courage to say it to your face! Here goes:

You will wonder why you had to suffer while others have such wonderful pregnancy experiences. Instead of feeling as though this is the worst thing that has ever happened to you, try thinking of it as the best thing that has ever happened to you (put that lighted match down!).

As new mothers we can't help but wonder what mistakes we'll make. Will we be good mothers, and how will we deal with the different challenges motherhood brings us? We HG sufferers know that when we deliver that precious child, we have won a huge battle! We are stronger then we ever imagined we could be. Realizing this about you is the best gift to receive when becoming a mother. We know we can endure and face with incredible strength anything that comes our way. We were put to the test early on and we passed! We do have what it takes to be great mothers, tough women, and strong human beings.

You will never take for granted the miraculous process of bringing a person into this world. You fought hard for that baby and you're a better person because of it. You will not take for granted those beautiful warm days and enjoying a meal with family and friends. You will appreciate little things, like cleaning your home, preparing foods, and enjoying the aroma that accompanies it. You will be grateful and truly know the value of being able to sit down with your kids and play with them. One of the first things I did when I came home from the hospital was to play with my son. You will cherish the time spent at gymnastic practices and basketball games. You are special and lucky to be able to look at life with new eyes and respect what it has to offer. You will be more optimistic then ever before and will be inspired to live every day to the fullest. From one HG sister to another: I applaud you!

How to help the HG sufferer

HG will affect not just the mother-to-be, but everyone who has a close bond with her. Your relationship will definitely be put to the test. Feelings will be hurt, insensitive and tactless remarks will be exchanged, and loved ones left feeling unappreciated. Marriage between the mother and father-to-be will take a beating. Just remember those important vows, "in sickness and in health." Be aware of what challenges lie ahead of you and don't forget that this too shall pass!

It's normal to feel helpless and frustrated as you watch your loved one suffer. Just know there are things you can do to help her. You aren't useless. In fact, you can be very instrumental in making this pregnancy go more smoothly. Here are some ways you can help her survive this pregnancy:

Share this Book with Her

When you finish reading this book, lend it to her. Better yet—read it to her. She may feel too ill to read, but can lie there and listen. Read only a few tips at a time and then afterwards take some time to understand and comprehend what you've read, letting her give your her opinions and feedback. Be sure to share your thoughts as well.

The fact that you've read to her shows you want to learn more about her condition and what goes along with it. It will show you care about her. Just hearing the testimonies will validate what she's feeling and what she's been trying to explain since she first began to feel bad. I constantly wanted to describe how I felt and I wouldn't stop until I felt the person truly understood what I was trying to explain. When I began reading the testimonies, I would insist my husband to read them and I would tell him, "That's exactly how I feel. I'm not the only one!" To me it was proof that I wasn't exaggerating or being a big baby about things. I wasn't just a wimp who couldn't handle being pregnant with a little "morning sickness." Even though I had been diagnosed with Hypermesis Gravidum long before, I always referred to it as morning sickness or nausea so others would know what I was talking about. After reading testimonies from others who'd gone through the same thing, I began referring to my sickness as HG. I didn't want others with the normal morning sickness telling me their experience and how they would "tough it out" at work. Anyone who truly has HG would never say it is possible to "tough it out."

When you're both finished with the book, give to someone else who's close to her and ask them to read some of the testimonies. If you've already lent the book out, then discuss with others what you read and learned. Remember to share anything you learn about HG, regardless of where or who you learned it from—this book, the Internet, her physician, or the mother herself. The word and education about HG needs to get out!

Ask Her How you Can Help

It can be that simple. Ask her what you can do to help her get through this. It may be hard for her to call upon you to do something for her. I know I absolutely dreaded asking for help of any kind. It was always much easier to accept someone's offer rather than having to ask them. The goal is to make this time for her as easy as possible. If she turns you down at first, don't hesitate to suggest your help again. If you continue to volunteer yourself to her, she will eventually realize you're sincere about wanting to help.

Keep in mind that if she was an independent woman before this sickness set in, then she needs to adjust to letting others do things for her. Consider your wording the next time you aim to lend a helping hand. For example, she will be more willing to request something from the store if it won't cause you to go out of your way.

"I need to go to the store today and pick up a few things. Is there anything I can pick up for you while I'm there?" Versus: "Would you like me to go to the store for you today?"

Although BOTH offers are fine and very considerate, the first suggestion might lead her to believe you won't be going too far out of your way to help her, since you have to go to the store anyway. The second suggestion might cause her to decline so you won't "go out of your way."

"Would you like me to cook you something and bring it over?" Versus: "I just made a big pot of vegetable soup and it's going to go to waste. I'm going to be on your side of town this afternoon, so I'll make a quick stop by your house and drop some off to you!"

Again, both suggestions are kind and considerate. The second suggestion will be easier for her to accept. She'll feel less guilty knowing you aren't "going to too much trouble" for her. I'll leave you with one more example:

"Thursday is my only day off; do you want me to baby-sit that day?" Versus: "I'm off work Thursday and I'd like to spend some time with Garrett. Would it be ok if I picked him up and brought him to my house for a little while?"

The first offer, although helpful, could leave her declining your help because it's your only day off and she doesn't want to impose babysitting on you. Remember she cares about you as well and doesn't want you babysitting on you only day off work. The second offer insinuates that not only do you volunteer, but you want to spend time with her child.

Try and keep in mind how hard it would be to depend so much on others.

Support Her

Listen. Be there for her when she needs to vent and talk about what she's going through. It can be challenging to sit through someone telling you how they are feeling without feeling you should give your advice on how to solve the problem. This isn't what you need to be doing. Just listen. That's all that is required of you. Let her talk, or cry, and then repeat back to her what she said in different words to let her know you understand what she's going through.

She may need to do this often. If you see she isn't opening up, then asks if she wants to talk and reassure her you'll be glad to listen. She should be letting this frustration out. Being a good listener can be more helpful then anything the doctor could prescribe!

Believe Her

Never doubt her sickness. Believe her and reassure her that you don't question her condition. Your disbelief can be devastating. If you question the state she's in, then it would be a good idea to do some research of your own. So you're better equipped to understand what she's going through.

It's crucial not to compare her with other pregnant women. It is not the same. I don't know how many my husband would compare me to different women in his family who were pregnant. They had their complaints, but still managed to work full-time. I tried to explain that if they truly had HG, it would be nearly impossible to work a full-time job. I tried making it clear to my husband that what his relatives were experiencing was morning sickness—not HG! My husband would retaliate with, "Well, maybe she just can handle it a little better."

If he only knew how this would hurt my feelings. I would then begin to question myself, Could I make myself get up and do more? Was I dramatizing a little bit? Because I didn't want him thinking I wasn't trying to get better, I'd make several different attempts to get up and accomplish something, but I would find myself feeling worse and would have to lie down.

It may get frustrating when you think she isn't trying to get better. Don't ever accuse her of this, because it could devastate her and leave her to feel she's alone. If all she can do is lie in bed, then let her. She obviously needs the rest. If you're concerned that she isn't getting enough exercise, suggest taking a walk. If she declines, don't fight her on this. She ultimately knows her body and whether she's physically up to it. This doesn't mean never suggest it again. Encourage her the next day to get out for a few minutes. Maybe she'll feel more up to it.

If she's constantly lying down and you question whether depression has kicked in, then contact her physician and tell him or her your concerns regarding her despair. Remember you're her advocate right now and she's depending on you. If the doctor doesn't seem too concerned make sure you're clear about what's going on. Before you make the phone call, make a list of the things you wish to discuss with him. It can be intimidating talking to a doctor, so make sure you're prepared.

Encourage her

She may need a pep talk every day—and sometimes maybe every hour. Try and stay positive for her. Remind her to take it one day at a time. Suggest different ideas she hasn't tried yet. Ask her to take a small walk with you. (But don't forget there's a fine line between nagging and encouraging). Suggest it to her and let her make her own decision whether she is up to it or not. When she declines, don't let it offend you' simply let it go and ask her again at a different time.

Organize Help

One of the hardest things for your loved one who is suffering from HG is to continuously ask for help. The first couple of favors I asked weren't too bad, but when you constantly need help it gets more and more difficult to call upon people. So to help save her from having to do this, take it upon yourself. Ask others for help.

It will be easier on you and everyone else if there's team effort. First off, you need to get the team together. Take it upon yourself to contact a group of her friends and family and ask them to come together on a certain day and time. If she belongs to a church family, ask that it be announced at church or printed in the church bulletin. Be sure to give all the important details and consider giving a phone number for those who can't make the meeting but would still like to help out. (This also might be a good time to request she be put on the prayer list.) If she belongs to any clubs or organizations, you might want to contact them as well. And don't forget her co-workers or classmates; the more the merrier. You can all meet for lunch or at someone's home. It's important to have a schedule ready at the meeting. The schedule should include a list of needs for the mom-to-be. This might include providing transportation for her, accompanying her to the doctor's office, preparing meals for her, house cleaning, laundry, babysitting, and simply giving her a call on a regular basis to see how she's coping. If several people come, then break up in pairs or committees and let them volunteer what services they're willing to provide.

Some might not have the time to help out, but want to contribute financially, which might help pay for some daycare or a cleaning service, or simply compensate for money that is not coming in because she can't work. Some might agree to send cards and notes with words of encouragement. Make clear to them that everything is appreciated. Sincere gratitude will inspire the giver to continue helping.

It's important for everyone to take turns in whatever they are doing. If her mother-in-law volunteers to cook supper for the family, she will soon need a break. Nine months is a long time and it will be easy for them to get burned out!

Research

It's important for you to research HG. Get on the Internet and type "Hyperemesis Gravidarum" into a search engine and you'll find information about this condition so many women are going through. While you're visiting these sites, read some of the testimonials they provide. Every experience is different and can be educational to others. There will also be testimonials from the mother's husbands and other loved ones who share their stories in hopes of helping others. These stories can be extremely beneficial to you. You'll be stunned at how similar your feelings and thoughts are to those of other caregivers. The mother isn't the only one who needs comfort and reassurance during this time. You need to be reminded that these nine months will end!

Take Care of Yourself

You might find yourself putting your own needs on the backburner as you try to give 100 percent to your loved one. Although this is heroic of you, it isn't good for either of you. To successfully take care of someone you must first take care of yourself. You need rest too. Taking on way too much will leave you exhausted long before she starts feeling better.

You must find time to get away by yourself, visit friends, and do something that gets your mind off the situation at home. This will help you refuel your energy and spirit. Taking care of a sick person is overwhelming and needs some interruption, or you might find yourself going down a steep hill toward depression. If you're seeing signs of depression within yourself, it's important to immediately contact your physician.

Here are some quotes that might uplift your spirits-

"Have a strong mind and a soft heart"—Anthony J. D'Angelo

"I think illness is a family journey, no matter what the outcome. Everybody has to be allowed to process it and mourn and deal with it in their own way."—Marcia Wallace

"Sympathy sees and says 'I'm sorry.' Compassion sees and says 'I'll help."—Anonymous

"He deserves paradise who makes his companions laugh."—Mohammed

"May I never get too busy in my own affairs that I fail to respond to the needs of others with kindness and compassion."—Thomas Jefferson

"The best exercise for good relationships is bending over backward."—unknown

"We are not primarily put on this earth to see through one another, but to see one another through."—Peter DeVries

"The best thing to do behind a person's back—is pat it."—unknown

Prepare meals

Food at this time is the HG sufferer's worst enemy. The one thing worse then eating food is preparing it or smelling it. Relieving her of this chore will be helpful beyond words. During this time it's important for her to eat what she can. Postpone battles about nutrition until she starts feeling a little better. Consuming a little food is better than no food at all!

Before cooking, remember to open the windows and turn on the exhaust fan to keep smells at a minimum. Also, it's best to keep cooking at a minimum for the time being. By that I mean, when cooking you should try doubling the recipes and freeze leftovers for later. Try using the microwave or grill out whenever possible. Take-out isn't a bad idea either; it eliminates cooking and clean up all together!

Make an effort not to get frustrated when you've taken time to prepare food and she only takes one bite. I can assure you right now she'd like nothing more than to sit there and enjoy every bite. More than likely she'll be worried that you worked so hard on dinner and will feel awful that she can't eat it. Put her mind at rest with words of understanding. Tell her you'll wrap it up and place it in the refrigerator and maybe she can try again later or eat it for lunch the next day.

If she complains about how it's cooked or criticizes you in any way, try and have broad shoulders. I guarantee she's lashing out because she feels sick and frustrated—not because of the dinner. Giver her time and then talk about it.

Be her advocate

Sometimes you may need to speak for her. This is especially true when she goes to her doctor's appointment. Be sure not to leave the doctor's office without informing her physician of her current condition. Don't sugarcoat it in any way.

Many times, during appointments with my doctor, I would tell him I was the same as last month. I would add that I wasn't throwing up as much, and then that would be about it. I should have told him that although I hadn't vomited as much, I was still extremely nauseated and felt miserable every day. I needed to tell him I felt like an emotional train wreck and was about to lose it. I'd wait weeks to get in to see him, just to say I was doing okay.

Now I realize I wasn't emotionally strong enough to go in there alone and tell him what I was really going through at home. I was afraid I would start crying if I tried to talk about it. So I didn't. I thought there was nothing he could do for me anyway, so why bother? Don't let your loved one go to her doctor with this attitude. Go with her and be her voice. Stand up for her, because she may be unable to do it herself. Tell the doctor what she's experiencing—and do not leave anything out. Address every concern you both have. Don't leave that office without having all your questions answered. You both should leave feeling a little better then when you got there. You both will have your chance to vent to the doctor and get his input, which might give you hope and encouragement to survive this HG!

Also defend her to others. If you hear someone talking about her condition in disbelief, then this is your chance to politely educate someone on HG. Maybe you can help mend wounds that were caused by the HG sufferer. There may be times when she lashes out at others. Make clear to them that she isn't herself right now and encourage them to remember what she's going through. Ask them not to hold grudges because this is a time when she needs them most.

Be considerate

Keep the toilet clean! I hesitated to add this because it seems like common sense, but sometimes people don't think of such things. Clean the toilet as often as possible. It's just as simple as that! Avoid eating in front of her. I cannot describe the love hate relationship with food your loved one is experiencing right now. She may desperately want to eat, but as soon as her favorite foods are placed in front of her she pushes it away and runs for the nearest restroom. She may say she isn't hungry, but that doesn't mean she wants to sit and watch you scarf down a juicy cheeseburger in front of her. Not to mention, the sight and smell of food may disgust her and add to her frustration. This isn't to say you can't eat for the duration of her sickness; just use a little tact at mealtime. If she's in the living room lying down, then be sure to eat in the kitchen. Keep your comments to yourself regarding how delicious the meal was!

Keep the smell down

Try not to wear your favorite cologne for a while—this will save her a trip to the bathroom! Also try to refrain from smoking anywhere near her, because the smell of smoke might worsen her nausea. The smell also might get on her clothes and stay with her for awhile, so stay clear when lighting up!

Also when buying detergent and fabric softener, shop for those that offer unscented. Ask her if hanging out the linen on the clothes line would leave a scent that would be too strong for her.

Eliminate noise

Noise can be extra annoying when you aren't feeling well. Take it from me, I'm the world's biggest TV junkie, but when I was sick the television drove me crazy. There were times when I could watch it, but it had to be the right time. Ask her if she'd like for you to sit in another room to watch your program. She may want you to stay in the room with her for company and sacrifice the silence. Let her make the decision!

Have a talk with the kids

Be sure to discuss with the kids how important it is to keep the commotion down during this time. Children will want to help, so give them this task. Siblings have their share of yelling matches and fights, but encourage them to keep it down and try to get along to help mom!

Treat her

Send her a card or some flowers. This will lift her spirits and remind her that she's special and cared about. If she's having a rare good day, then take her for a manicure or give her a foot rub.

I remember getting a few cards in the mail and, on one occasion, flowers. It was so surprising because most were from people I didn't have a close relationship with. Some of the cards came from people I'd only spoken with a few times. The fact that these people took time to not only think of me but send a card wishing me well totally blew me away. I was so touched and I learned a great deal from these people. I never was one who put a lot of effort in greeting cards of any kind. I thought they were a waste of money. But I learned cards are very powerful and can truly bring inspiration and comfort to the one who receives them. It's a small gesture that can make a huge difference.

Testimonies

I wanted to share my story because I wanted you to have the perspective of someone with a less severe form of this affliction.

Right now I am 11 weeks pregnant with my second baby. I had "mild" HG with my first pregnancy, but this time I would say it is more "moderate" in nature. I have to tell you that even mild to moderate cases are extremely debilitating. Like many of the more severe HG sufferers, I am on Zofran and Phenergan. But, despite the medication I still vomit occasionally. More often than not, I just spend hours in front of the toilet trying to vomit, but with just a really bad case of the dry heaves. Even though dry heaving isn't as bad, it still prevents you from eating and getting proper hydration, which is a problem. I am not in the hospital (yet). I haven't lost any weight; in fact, I have gained five pounds. But, for me every day is different. Here is what has happened to me:

1. **I have lost the ability to care about myself and others.** Even though I am nauseous every day, some days are much worse than others and it is completely unpredictable. Some days are so bad that I have to rely on the kindness of my mother, sister, or husband just to make sure that my 18 month old gets fed and gets her diapers changed. I feel like I have lost the ability to care for myself, my daughter, my dogs and my house. I can't even cook! Which is sort of ironic, because if you can't cook, you can't eat, and if you don't eat something, the nausea is usually worse? On "good" days, small feats are major accomplishments, like paying bills, taking a shower, ordering groceries online, giving my daughter a bath, or going out in public.

2. **I have become socially withdrawn.** Going out in public is scary when you have HG. Generally, I don't do it, unless my husband or mom is with me. And when I'm really nauseous, I avoid it altogether. I mean, imagine going to the park or grocery store, and you start to get that nauseous feeling. You know, clammy hands, rapid pulse, stomach churning, etc. All the sudden you realize you have to vomit, but don't make it to a toilet. So now you have just vomited in front of

an audience. I can just picture it, my daughter would start to cry because she gets scared when I vomit, and strangers surround you offering help that they can't give. What a nightmare!!! During my first pregnancy, my husband had made a comment to me that he wondered if the "old me" was ever going to come back. He couldn't understand why I didn't want to hang out with friends or go to restaurants, etc. This just made me cry. He is a good husband. He loves me and he's helpful. But when he doesn't even understand, how is anyone else going to?

3. **I can't help it, but I hate everyone**! Everyone is just so darn uninformed. Even when people offer well-intentioned suggestions, they really make me mad. Even the nurses at my ob-gyn, who should know better, are suggesting lemon water, crackers, and ginger ale. It's like being treated like you have the sniffles when you have the full-blown flu or pneumonia. Another thing that drives me nuts is everyone telling me I will be over it soon. When I tell people I had nausea through 16 weeks in my first pregnancy I get reactions like "Oh my God!" Actually, according to the hyperemesis.org website, 50% of women still experience nausea and vomiting at 14 weeks. By 20 weeks it drops off to 10%. But still, it is a giant myth that this magically disappears at the beginning of the second trimester.

4. **The first part is because of the way I feel; this will be my last baby.** It makes me sad, But I can't just rely on my 60 year old mother to take care of me and my child for weeks on end because I am vomiting. And based on the other stories people have shared, my next pregnancy could be worse. Knowing that is enough to say this is it.

Lisa

Having HG has given me a new perspective on life. Before my pregnancy I was a healthy active adult. After becoming pregnant I was debilitated by a horrible disease that literally made me feel like I was going to die. I am currently 32 weeks pregnant with my first child. I was diagnosed with HG at 8 weeks, by my first doctor. She tried treating me with all the HG drugs: Reglan, all forms of Zofran. I worried a lot, none of the medications seemed to help and even though I was assured that these drugs were safe in pregnancy, I was taking them in such large doses that I was afraid ten years from now a new study would come out and reveal those levels did in fact cause some horrible childhood illness. At the end of my first trimester I had not gained any weight, lost my job, and had been hospitalized four times for dehydration. The stress was really getting to me. My doctor then suggested that I go on the Zofran pump. The home health care nurse came out and for the first time I truly felt like I might die. Here I wanted a natural birthing experience, but instead I was forced to jab myself every other day to receive medication that was costing me over $500 a day. The stress was overwhelming and I found myself in the hospital again, this time not for dehydration but for having a severe panic attack at 3:00 in the morning. My husband thought I had finally gone crazy. He stopped talking about having a second child! I sought out a specialist almost 800 miles away in order to receive better medical care; I was not going to let this disease harm myself or my child. I really thought I would lose the baby, I was finishing my second trimester and still had not gained one pound-I was lucky just to be vomiting 4 or 5 times a day instead of the 16–18 times without the Zofran pump. The specialist immediately admitted me into the hospital. While I was there I received a whole round of physicals and went through IV hyper alimentation. It has been three weeks now since I was in the hospital and at my last check up I had gained nine pounds. It turns out my HG was furthered by having horrible acid reflux, now all I take is Zantac, and occasionally a Zofran ODT if I feel really nauseated. We are now in the process of moving so the doctor who helped me overcome my HG can deliver my baby and be her pediatrician. I do not know how I could have continued on without his help.

Emaandamy

HG has been most excruciating and frustrating experience I have ever had to go through. Even though you have family and friends trying to be supportive mostly they can be non-motivating because they cannot possibly know what it's like for you at the time you are suffering.

My HG is not severe, I do not lose weight, I actually gain too much of it and I think I do this as a survival mechanism and also as an attempt to comfort me through the depression that I suffer from the constant nausea. Through my first pregnancy I had to suffer in silence as my doctors (military) would not prescribe any meds for my condition. They pretty much just told me to suck it up and that it was just part of being pregnant. So I suffered from daily and constant unrelenting nausea for the whole pregnancy and vomited at least twice a day. But still managed to gain 50 plus pounds. Now I don't know if there are any other women out there who gain weight during this time, but I would sure like to hear from them as well.

I am now 34 weeks with my second child and I have a much better experience this time around. I found a civilian doctor who is very understanding to my needs and he right away diagnosed me with HG and prescribed me **Zofran.** This drug is a miracle drug and since I have been on it I have not suffered like I did with my first. I am much more peaceful and excited about my pregnancy than I was with my first one.

I hope a lot more doctors listen to their patients and a lot more insurance companies cover this drug for women who suffer from this condition even if it is not that severe. I cannot even think about how I would be feeling right now if I did not have this drug to help me cope.

So this is my survival story and I am still surviving and just taking this all one day at a time.

Starmoons1220

I am currently 38 weeks pregnant and I was diagnosed with HG at 9 weeks. I went from not having any nausea to throwing up anything and everything (including small portions of saltines and water) within a matter of only two weeks. I also became severely depressed because many people told me I was overreacting. I knew that something was wrong; I knew I must have more than the usual morning sickness. Still, most people didn't believe me. At my lowest point, I was hugging the toilet, sobbing, and actually thinking that death might be a better option than having children. After vomiting so often (to the extent of vomiting bile and then "dry-heaving" when nothing was left), I became so weak and dehydrated that I could not stand up without nearly fainting. When all was said and done, I had lost about 12 pounds and a week of work.

Since I had been treated by a doctor for fertility issues and then switched to a midwife in his practice after becoming pregnant, there was a mix-up when I first called the office for advice (late on a Sunday evening). Instead of contacting the midwife, the answering service had my former doctor return my call. I had not been able to keep down anything for almost 48 hours, and he literally suggested a "clear liquid diet"—nothing but popsicles, Gatorade, and water. He did not ask if I had lost any weight, and he said that this was plain old morning sickness. Worst of all, he talked down to me like I was just wasting his time. By the next morning, I had not slept for almost 48 hours and was now even retching when I tried to sip Gatorade.

I decided to call the office again, and I got in touch with one of my midwives. She was very upset with the doctor's lack of concern, and she assured me that she would be more vigilant—since I had already lost so much weight and become so weak. She immediately called in a prescription for Promethazine (Phenergan) and said to get back to her if I could not hold down the medication. She said that it might become necessary to give me a suppository form of the medication or to hospitalize me if my condition would not stabilize on the oral meds. She also warned me that I would likely be sleepy, but said that I should be able to eat "bland foods" again by that evening-though I should probably stick to Gatorade a few more hours while the drug kicked in.

I thought I must have died and gone to heaven! By that evening, I was actually able to eat some solid food—and I didn't even throw it back up. A few days later, I was capable of moving around the house without assistance, and I was eating and drinking normal foods without vomiting. In the next few weeks, I slowly gained back the weight I had lost, and I went back to work without a problem.

When I reached my second trimester, the midwife suggested I try to wean myself off the medication; she said that many women stop experiencing morning sickness at about that time. Unfortunately, I was not one of those women. Although I was able to function very well on only one dose of Promethazine per day, I rapidly deteriorated when I stopped taking the drug all together. After another month, I decided to try again—but to no avail. It seemed that I would be on this drug "forever," and a lot of people were putting pressure on me to "stop taking unnecessary medication." When I voiced my concerns to my midwife, she reassured me by stating that these people were not trained medical professionals and didn't know any better. My midwife also told me something else that really helped to ease my conscience—taking the medication was the one thing that made my body capable of holding down the nutrients my body needed to form a healthy baby.

Although some people still don't seem to understand why I am taking drugs for HG, I no longer care what they think. Unless you have suffered from HG, you frankly cannot understand. Crissy

I'm in my second (and right now I am certain, my last) pregnancy, and trying to get through day by day with HG. I had it during my first pregnancy, suffered miserably until 10 weeks when I was given Zofran. This helped tremendously. This time, as soon as I developed symptoms (nausea all day, everyday) I called my OB and requested Zofran. I am taking it twice a day, but I still feel so crummy. I know it is helping at least a little because I am at least able to eat some foods in very small portions, but I still FEEL terrible all day long. I also feel depressed and isolated, as I am home all day alone with no help taking care of my two year old (my husband works long hours). The worst part is that you feel like nobody really understands. People say, Oh, your having some morning sickness, huh?" and I want to strangle them. Morning sickness implies that after the morning, it goes away ... no such luck. The only person in my life who understands is my grandma, because she went through it with all three of her pregnancies. And they didn't have Zofran or any medications for it back then. They treated her as if it were a psychiatric condition, telling her that she brought it on herself and was trying to get attention. Can you imagine! They even had her evaluated by a psychiatrist, asking her questions like "Do you resent your baby? Do you resent your husband? She said it was the most demeaning experience of her life. So, I try to be grateful that I live in a time where at least some doctors recognize it as a real condition and there are some treatments available. Meanwhile, I take it one day at a time. I am now nine weeks, and I know that it will likely let up around 12–14 weeks (as it did in my first pregnancy), but that is no consolation right now. Each day, hour, minute is misery. I won't do this again. I know it sounds selfish, but this is my last pregnancy if I have any say over it. I just can't physically or emotionally go through this again.

Charliebenny

The nine months I suffered from hyperemesis were the worst months of my life but I made it through and got the most wonderful, precious gift. I might be crazy but I am actually thinking about having another. I know I will probably be sick again but I now know the reward outweighs the suffering.

I had hyperemesis for my entire pregnancy; my daughter is now 14 months and perfectly healthy. I lost a total of thirty pounds, was on all sorts of medications (zofran, raglan, phenergan) including steroids AND had gall bladder surgery when I was five months pregnant. I too was extremely worried about the weight loss and being on so many medications for nausea plus morphine after the surgery. I am happy to say that I gave birth to a healthy baby who weighed 8lbs. 11oz. The doctor kept telling me she was getting what she needed from my stored fat and apparently she was right. My doctor said I was the worst pregnancy she had ever been a part of. Hang in there. I know how it feels, like it will never end but I can tell you that it was all worth it once I had my beautiful baby and I would do it again.

Aims19

In 1995 I became pregnancy and at nine weeks I was throwing up nonstop for twenty-four hours. I was basically sick both ways. I did not know what was wrong with me other than that I was extremely sick. At first I went to Urgent Care. I ended up having such a bad experience there with an on-call doctor. First, he did not want to treat me with an IV and then he told me he is not good at getting the IV's in. When he finally did get the IV in, he thought I was making myself throw up. The sickness got worse and later that night I was admitted to the hospital his final words from him and nurse were "don't eat anything for a week." I was on bedrest and so sick throughout the entire pregnancy. I ended up going to the hospital 40 times for the pregnancy and was induced at 36.5 weeks. I was told I was the worst case they had ever seen. I dealt with all this while having an alcoholic husband. My funniest night (if you can call any of this funny) was when I was admitted to the hospital and I had to share a room. The poor girl I was sharing a room with couldn't even take a shower as I was throwing up all night. While I lay there dying in my bed, (she was scheduled to have a C-section the next day) I got the pleasure of having her and her husband's pizza delivery guy walk by me. That was great fun. Then, the nurses made me eat some Turkey Wild Rice Soup. I warned them that I would throw it all up but they didn't believe me. Sure enough it was all over everything. I survived and had a beautiful son.

In 2002, I remarried and we lost our first baby in May 2004 (miscarriage) and then had to terminate in November 2004. I had been to the hospital for vomiting and was on home-care but it was just so horrible and painful I couldn't even swallow a bowl of soup. We are in the process of adopting with American Adoptions and then we will try again and face HG hell again in two years. I will have a little more challenges my nine year old son, my sister lives with us who has Down's Syndrome she is 51, and came to live with us three years ago when my mom died, and then the baby I adopt. I am praying and trying to prepare myself for HG this time. It is horrendous and unfair but all you can do is managing it the best you can. Thank-you for reading my story.

Elizabeth

With my first pregnancy I was diagnosed with HG when I was roughly five weeks along. I lost a lot of weight and was extremely dehydrated before my doc's prescribed Diclectin. That medication did take the edge of the nausea but that's all. The HG continued to get worst until it peaked at about 5–6 months. I got to the point where I couldn't bring myself to swallow food. I would try ... I'd chew and chew and roll it around in my mouth and would have to force myself to swallow. Did not seem to matter what type of food or if I liked it or not.

People around me had little or no sympathy. They just kept saying it's just morning sickness and soon I'd be feeling better. I still harbor ill feelings toward those people. I remember I was telling my sister-in-law of my sickness when my mother-in-law came in the room. My sister-in-law asked my mother-in-law if it was really that bad. Standing right beside me she said, "No it's not really that bad." I was floored. I understand that she has not had kids yet and we don't want to frighten her but hey!!! Yes it really can be that bad!

The diclectin made it so that I could keep at least one meal down per day (still throwing up about 4–6 times a day.) I did not gain much weight in the end but still managed to be within the norm by the end. I was sick every day for the full pregnancy. I tried several times to go off the medication but when I did I was not even able to keep water down.

It took a long time before I could accept the risk of another pregnancy. I just could not shake the feeling that I wanted to have just one more. Suffering from endometriosis spurred on my decision. Once I got pregnant again and 4 weeks in began feeling the sickness coming on again I began to question my sanity. I also have a ruptured disk in my lower back and of course all the vomiting aggravated it severely. I was useless to anyone and landed myself in the hospital after not keeping food down for three days. The dilectin seemed like it was not working at all this time. As I live in Canada that is all they were willing to give me (for at home use). I was afraid to leave the hospital as I felt I'd just have to turn around and come back again. A couple of weeks after that I had my first ultrasound and found out that I am carrying twins!! That might explain why the meds are not working so well this time.

I have been in the hospital two more times since then—the last stay was five days. They had a lot of trouble getting my electrolytes to balance. My potassium was very low despite all their efforts. They also discovered I have a heart murmur they think due to the stress of the pregnancy. I am currently 19 weeks along and still throwing up regularly. I don't expect this will get better until I give birth. I just hope I can get enough nutrition to support two babies. They sure are not leaving much for me.

In the beginning, every minute seems like a fight fir survival. I have been lucky that my struggle reduced to hourly and now daily. You really feel like someone has poisoned you and that you no longer have the means of digesting food. The fact that so few people understand that this is a real condition, we are not faking and we do not have eating disorders. I had people who hated me because I put on so little weight in my pregnancy, but they just don't understand that I would have gladly gained the weight than to be throwing up for that long.

I needed lots of dental work after having my little girl and I lost about 30% of my hair. Not looking forward to that again. My meds are expensive too and I sure don't have the extra $200 per month but what can you do? It's either that or never leave the hospital.

Sorry about the rambling and venting!
Deb

Hello there … oh my goodness where do I start … first off let me thank you for wanting to write a book about this subject, it would have been a comfort to read about other people's experiences when I went through HG. I had HG with my first pregnancy…. everything was going fine up until about my 8th week…. then the nausea hit—it was constant and never went away…. as a week passed things got worse I started throwing up about three times a day (which made going to work and taking public transit a real problem)…. eventually I became so ill I was afraid to leave my house for fear of vomiting in public…. by this time I had to quit my job and my mother-in-law came to get me to stay with her until I was feeling better (I couldn't get off the sofa to take care of even my most basic needs)…. well about a week into staying with my mother-in-law it got worse, I was throwing up every twenty minutes…. they admitted me into the hospital where they had me on an IV of Gravol and giving me diclectin…. I stayed from 12 weeks to my 18th week…. by this time I had lost 30 pounds…. I still felt ill throughout the remainder of my pregnancy…. I took gravol and diclectin everyday…. by the time I was full term I still weighed less than what I did before I was pregnant…. Luckily, I had a healthy baby girl, she is now 2 and doing great.

Kim

Hi,

I have suffered through the hell that is hyperemesis with two pregnancies so far. With my first daughter Lili I was sick for 20 weeks. It feels like to me I have poison running through my body when I get pregnant. With my first pregnancy, I had a doctor who kept telling me, "this is normal, all women go through it"—normal to be throwing up 37 times (yes I counted) a day, dry heave for 2 hours straight, pass out on the bathroom floor, lose 22 ponds in two months while pregnant, be so badly dehydrated that my lips were cracked and bleeding, and still he said it's normal-keep taking your B, we do not prescribe any anti nausea medications here. Well somehow I made it through, and delivered my beautiful daughter Lili.

After that I waited three years to try again, out of fear of the hyperemesis, but this time I did some research and picked a doctor that specialized in helping Hyperemesis patients, and was a lot more sympathetic to it. With my second pregnancy, the hyperemesis started at 4 ½ weeks, he prescribed phenergan which I took every 4 hours, which took a slight edge off, but by week 6, no longer worked anymore. This time I could not eat anything, or drink any liquid, the moment liquid hit my stomach, I would vomit profusely, every time I moved, go up (which is a lot when you have to take care of a three year old) I would vomit sometimes on her. He then prescribed Zofran, which did not help me at all. I finally had to go into the hospital for four weeks straight, and lay in a dark room, on an IV where I did not eat or drink for weeks. Even turning on a light made me sick. If I made the smallest movement, or smelled anything at all, I would vomit. I can honestly say there were moments that I entertained dying rather than going on another moment like this, but the daughter and the new baby kept me going. With this pregnancy, I lost 18 pounds in the first two months. Unfortunately, after all this suffering I lost the baby at 16 weeks, he turned out to be sick and there was nothing they could do. I felt so cheated; I had done all this for nothing and put my daughter through so much. Then I had all this guilt about taking all those medications in huge doses. They say it's safe but who really knows for sure (my baby had a chromosome problem; I did not lose him to the medications.)

My husband till this day admits that he could not go through what I went through for anything in the world. Our problem now is we still want another child. I just don't know if I can live through it again. I know it is worth it in the long run, but I am terrified.

For all the women who have suffered though this out there, you are brave, strong, unselfish women, and I commend you. It is probably one of the most difficult things to go through; at least it is worth it in the end.

Susie

Nine years ago I had my first HG pregnancy. I did not know there was a name for it. I didn't even know anyone else got that sick during pregnancy. I was told (and I believed) that it was all in my head. NO ONE gets that sick during pregnancy. During that pregnancy I had to quit my job because I couldn't work. It took me seven years to forget how bad it was.

Seven years later I decided I wanted another child bad enough that I would try it again. I believed every pregnancy was different and that this one wouldn't be as bad. Well, it wasn't as bad, but it was still very tough. I remember lying in bed because I couldn't move anymore due to nausea and crying because I felt like a terrible mother because I just didn't want to be pregnant anymore. I was miserable. After that pregnancy, my husband and I decided that was it. I couldn't go through it again. Just when I had come to terms with this decision, we found out we were pregnant again.

I cried for hours when I found out. I love my son, but I did not want to go through another pregnancy again. I was right. That pregnancy was the worst of all. At about eleven weeks, I began throwing up and not being able to stop. I wound up admitted to the hospital for two days. Two weeks later, I was in the ER for fluids. Two weeks after that I was in the doctor's office getting fluids by IV. The day after I returned to work from the episode I was fired. I was not able to return to work until after my son was born. Five weeks after his birth I was back to work full time. If we had not been able to borrow money from our parents during the time I was sick, we would almost definitely have lost our house and probably our vehicles. I was also unable to care for my then 11 month old. She had to continue attending daycare the whole time I was out of work. I had read many stories of women who had much worse cases of HG and my heart goes out to them again and again. I know how terrible I felt through mine, and I don't wish that on anyone.

With my last pregnancy, after getting fluids in the ER I received an instruction sheet on how to treat Hyperemesis. I was so excited. What I suffered from had a name. Then I found the HER website. Without that website, I don't know what would have happened. I was at the point in my pregnancy where I was seriously considering terminating. Without the support from the HER website, I don't know if I would have gone through with that or not. I thank GOD every time I look at my son that I found that site when I did.

Wendy

I'm a 37 year old Canadian living in Australia, married to an Australian. After struggling to become pregnant for some time and then finally conceiving on my second cycle of IVF, my husband and I were so happy and thrilled. We were on such a high. Finally, my hardships and struggles with infertility and IVF were over and we were going to be parents. We expected the pregnancy to be a happy and exciting time, free of any problems, because after all, we figured that we had already paid our dues! How could we have been so wrong!

After a week of bliss, it began. I woke up one morning feeling so very nauseous. It was a strange sort of nausea as it never went away. I've always been the sort of person that hated being nauseated and vomiting more than anything. It always scared me so much.

After weeks, the vomiting began. It was nonstop. Every fifteen minutes. I was given ginger, vitamin B6 injections, Stemetil suppositories and Maxalon. Nothing helped. By the next weekend I went into the hospital for IV. First of several visits. I was dumbfounded and couldn't understand what was happening to me. Surely this wasn't typical "morning sickness"? I was also becoming angry and depressed. All my friends were getting pregnant on their first attempts, or so they said, and were having wonderful pregnancies. God must have been punishing me for something. I also became very angry with God.

For my second visit to a hospital, I went to a different hospital. It paid off. They gave me Zofran. It helped for a while to reduce the vomiting. However, I didn't know I could increase the dosage. Anyway, the vomiting got worse again. A couple of more trips to the hospital for IV and dealing with ignorant and rude medical staff. Fortunately, my husband is very strong and was able to battle for me. He wasn't going to put up with any mistreatment. You need someone to bat for you in these situations.

The struggles continued. The Zofran caused constipation at times I thought was worse than the vomiting. Then it occurred to me. I could end my suffering by either terminating my pregnancy or by killing myself. I was so depressed. I had no support except my husband who was at work. You see, all my family is in Canada. I booked an appointment for an abortion. My husband said he'd divorce me if I went through with it. So I ended up canceling my appointment the night before for fear of having to go through it all alone.

I went back into the hospital for a week where they kept a close eye on me and organized for a psychologist to visit me regarding my frequent panic attacks and suicidal thoughts. I was so scared of throwing up just one more time that I'd have an actual panic attack. Anyway, they increased my dosage of Zofran and gave me Ranitidine. I seemed to stabilize.

My mother then came out from Canada for ten weeks to nurse me back to health. Eventually, the nausea started easing and by around 22 weeks I had only mild nausea which lasted the duration of the pregnancy. I gave birth by C-section to a beautiful baby girl, Rachel Emilie. She was so worth it all.

Having suffered fertility problems, our methods of contraception weren't that great and I was shocked to find myself pregnant again when my first was only 10 months old. I totally freaked out! I cried hysterically. I was so terrified of going through HG again. Once again my life would be turned upside down.

Fortunately, we were experienced this time and I was able to get onto Zofran much earlier. As a result, I didn't get quite as the first time. This time I tried acupuncture, but it didn't work. I also was given Droperidol while in the hospital which helped a lot. I also found that sniffing peppermint oil helped take the edge off the nausea. My mother couldn't come out from Canada this time as she was going through chemotherapy for colon cancer and my father was very sick with Alzheimer's disease. I certainly had a lot on my mind and became depressed again. Fortunately, a friend of mine flew out from Canada and stayed with us for a while and helped care for me and my toddler. As the depression became quite severe, my GP paid me some home visits and ended up prescribing me the antidepressant Mertazapine. It has also been known to help with nausea. Well, the next day the nausea was almost completely gone. It was amazing! I continued to suffer mild nausea for the remainder of my pregnancy and took Zofran and Mertazapine, but it was totally manageable. Unfortunately, my emotional trials were far from over. My father passed away while I was seven months pregnant and I was unable to fly back to Canada to be with my family and for the funeral. It was an awful year. On the bright side, I gave birth by C-section to a healthy, beautiful baby girl, Jessica Hope.

Jessica is now nine months old and doing really well. My mother has finished chemotherapy and seems to have beaten the cancer. I still suffer flashbacks to those awful early days of my pregnancies. Sometimes I lie in bed and can't sleep as I relive those experiences in my mind. I also suffer many food aversions. I wonder if the nightmares will ever go away. On the bright side, I have two beautiful little girls who bring me much joy. Oh, I also had a tubal ligation. So definitely no more HG for me.

Good luck to all of you who are suffering HG. Hang in there. Please, please make sure you are getting the help and support you need. It's so important, and can make all the difference.

HG Survivor in Australia
Judy

People ask me to describe HG and I always say, **"Imagine waking up from the worst hangover ever. The kind where you make a deal with God never to drink again because you feel so bad. Now imagine waking up and feeling that way 24/7 for your ENTIRE pregnancy."**

I am an HG survivor. I have two children. My daughter is 2 ½ and my son is 4 months. I had HG with both pregnancies. I had SEVERE HG with my son.

I knew I was pregnant with my son at about 5 weeks. I was hospitalized the first time for IV when I was 8 weeks pregnant. I was in and out of the hospital for IV treatment during weeks 9–12 of my pregnancy. I spent 12 days in the hospital for week 13. I took every drug to try to help with the nausea. I took Zofran, Reglan, and Compazine. Nothing helped. I lost 22 lbs. the first three months.

I was in the pit of depression. I had thoughts of suicide. I'm embarrassed to say there were times when I hoped I would have a miscarriage. This 2nd baby was planned and I wanted to have another child, but I could not take the nausea or the vomiting.

There were days when I just didn't want to wake up. I would cry the moment I got up because it was another day of HG that I had to face.

My sense of smell was heightened. I was able to smell everything. My husband would open a can of Pepsi, and I could smell it from the next room.

There were days when I could not get up from bed. I had a bucket next to me because I could not make it to the bathroom. There were days, sometimes even weeks where I would be wearing the same clothes. I could hardly take a shower. The smell of the soap or shampoo would make me throw up. I would gag every time I tried to brush my teeth. I would vomit every time after I brushed my teeth.

On good days, when I could make it to the bathroom, I would spend my day lying on the cold tile floor. I would think to myself, "Why is my body betraying me like this?"

Not only couldn't I keep anything down (including water) every time I threw up, I would wet my pants.... every single time. I can laugh about it now, but at the time, it was humiliating.

I spent the summer of 2005, laying in bed, with the air conditioner on full blast and in total darkness. I couldn't speak, eat, drink, or talk. On the rare occasion that I would watch TV, it seems that every commercial was about food. I had this awful taste in my mouth all the time. I was constantly spitting. So in between the vomiting, wetting myself, I had to spit. Since my husband is a teacher, he had the summer off and was able to care for our daughter. He was patient and he tried to understand but it was difficult for him to really comprehend what I was going through.

I was so jealous when I would go to my doctors and see other pregnant women. They looked so happy. They were actually ENJOYING being pregnant. I was jealous:

1. For the cravings they had

2. of their "pregnancy glow"

3. That they could enjoy this once in a lifetime experience

4. They didn't have to worry about finding a place to vomit AND pee at the same time.

People, who don't experience HG, can never understand what it is like. My grandmother would say, "I just can't sympathize with you. I was never ever sick for all 5 of my pregnancies."

I had HG for my entire pregnancy. I even threw up when I was in labor. When my son came out (via c-section) the second he left my body.... I was starving! I never experienced a hunger like that. Since I had a c-section, I was only allowed liquids, but I would have done anything for a burger with onion rings and a large coke!

Even though I had HG with both pregnancies, my daughter came in at 10 lbs. 1 oz, and my son was 8lbs. 4 oz. I often wonder if I had not been vomiting the whole time, would they have weighed even more.

I made the difficult decision of getting my tubes tied. I tried to think of it as.... "Well, I have my girl and my boy. I don't need anymore." But I would have liked to have had the option. HG robbed me of that. HG breaks your spirit. It tests your faith.

Take care and good luck!
Lisa

Hi!

I am a survivor of HG! I became pregnant with my first daughter when I was 21 years old. Within three weeks of becoming pregnant I became ill. Just a little nauseated at first and within another week I was violently ill. I could not keep down even a sip of water. One morning while I was still in bed my husband cracked an egg in the kitchen (which was on the other end of our house) and I could smell it!!! He thought I was crazy! I was hospitalized several times for dehydration and I was unable to work for three months. I told my husband that if he loved me he would kill me to put me out of my misery. I was very serious—I really wanted to die so that the suffering would end.

Four months into my pregnancy, I was still very nauseated and vomited sometimes, but I was able to function. I returned to work (at that time my husband and I worked together.) We had to pass a Mc Donald's on the way and every morning he would have to stop so I could throw up on the road. I did not eat at Mc Donald's for over a year after giving birth. When I did vomit there was very little warning—it just came up. This led to some very embarrassing moments of throwing up in my plate—once at a restaurant. A doctor actually came over because he thought I was dying.

Two weeks before my due date the nausea once again was severe. I could not keep anything down and I actually thought that I would never feel normal again. I had in my mind that I had developed some weird form of Bulimia.

I gave birth November 11, 1992 to Mallory. I had gained 6 pounds and she weighed 8lbs 5oz! I swear within two hours I felt like I could have ran a marathon. I had never felt better in my life! I ate everything I could get my hands on! In fact I didn't see what the big deal was about giving birth. I said and still say it was the easiest part of pregnancy for me. It meant that the suffering was almost over and my reward was on its way—literally.

I did not think I would ever do it again, but I did—two more times. Each time was a little worse and plus I had my children to care for. It is definitely worth every bit of suffering but when you are going through it—it is hell! I have been able to encourage a younger friend of mine who also suffered. I would like to help anyone that I can by sharing my story. I felt so alone and like no one understood and like I was some kind of freak. My family was supportive but I always felt like they thought it was in my head. They told me if I just would get up and get out I would feel better! People who haven't been through it just can't understand.

I hope that my story can encourage someone. Thank you for putting something together—I wish I had something I could have read. I had the book, "What to Expect…." and I would read the small one or two paragraphs over and over again—just to validate that I wasn't crazy and I wasn't alone.

Thanks again,
Kristy

I have always wanted to be a mom. I always loved children and knew they were an important part of my life. I am a teacher, and I can't express to you how much I love my job. Two years ago I became pregnant with our first child. My husband and I were absolutely thrilled. I knew that I would get nausea and vomiting, due to the fact that both my mom and sister were ill. My mom weighed the same amount when she went in to deliver, as she did before she was pregnant. I didn't realize how ill I would be. There was no hiding the illness. I couldn't even hold up my head. I vomited uncontrollably, bursting blood vessels in my eyes, nose and back of my throat. The nausea was horrific. The awful smells prevented me from leaving the house and that terrible over salivation. It dehydrated me even more. I had many, many trips to the hospital. Nothing seemed to help. No one knew what to do, and no one knew why I was SO ill. I had never heard of HG nor did any doctor ever tell me that this is what I had. My OB basically told me that I would die, and it was basically a mental thing. I lost 27 pounds and felt totally defeated. I turned into a ghostly shell. After 4 months I lost the baby. I was just so relieved that the illness was over. No more trips to the hospital. I could resume my normal life. My husband and I decided that we would remain childless. I would have all the lovely children that I taught. What more did I need. There was a great sadness on both sides of the family, especially my husband's mom, who was a former maternity nurse.

After a while, I found the HER website. I started to research. I wrote BC women's hospital and went in for an information session. I spent many many hours thinking about HG, and I finally understood why I was so ill. I also found others who were like me. I was not a freak, nor making it up in my mind, after all. I found a new OB, who was supportive. I developed a protocol, and prepared family and friends with information booklets. The maternal instinct took over and my husband and I tried again to make it through a pregnancy.

It happened very fast. I became ill very quickly! This time around, I was ready. I knew what I needed. My husband became my advocate. I was not able to hold up my head, or get off the bathroom floor for many moths. I was off work for six moths on a sick leave. I had all the horrible symptoms that I did before. This time when I went to the doctor he asked me what I needed, and I gave him my protocol. Zofran helped me get through the worst times. Along with gravol, and many other meds. More importantly though, the ladies on the forum knew and understood what was going on. Most importantly, my husband became a saint. He would wash out my disgusting spit buckets, cook his food on the BBQ outside in the middle of the Canadian winter, and held my head when I puked. He helped me live. He helped me survive. I developed SPD which is a separation in my pelvis. The HG lasted the full nine moths. I was vomiting and pushing on the delivery table. I was induced a day after my 40th week. The doctor discovered protein in my urine and I was swelling like a balloon. I also had a calcification on my placenta that was discovered on week31. On March 30, 2006 I gave birth to a beautiful baby girl. I had 20 hours of labor. She definitely was not ready to come. She was very far up. I had two epidurals that didn't take and ended up with numerous holes in my spine. The blood refused to clot in the holes and the spinal fluid was leaking in and out of the holes. I started to get spinal headaches. I had second degree tearing and an episiotomy. Many stitches and a forceps delivery. Nothing compared to the nausea I experienced for nine months. Gracee River Garrett was born weighing in at a healthy seven pounds, eleven ounces. My husband is absolutely smitten, and I am over the moon. I cry a lot, when I think of how lucky I am. I love every minute with her. I posted her birth story under the birth announcements.

I had a friend tell me;
When you lose a baby the spirit lives on, until you try again. The same spirit comes through each time, until it managed to get through into our world. This helped me realize that perhaps I didn't lose my baby after all the first time. She is here with me today. It just took her a little while to join us.

Carla

I suffered from HG from the time I found out I was pregnant (about 5 weeks) until 1 week after I delivered. I had to go to the ER 8 times to be rehydrated and 2 times I was admitted for overnight stays. I lost 15lbs my first trimester and only gained about 15 over my pre-pregnancy weight. About half way through my second trimester, I had a PICC line put in my arm. I had it for about two months. I was on oral Reglan and Lorazapam. I had IV Zofran when I had my PICC line. I could barely eat anything the whole time. My husband went crazy, and without him, I don't think I would have eaten at all. Mostly, I lived off of peanut butter and jelly sandwiches and chicken noodle soup (which I haven't eaten since, and its been 5 months) I cried everyday and wished I had never gotten pregnant. I wanted to strangle any person who told me to just eat crackers. Like I hadn't tried that!!! Crackers taste like glue when you have no spit in your mouth because you are so dehydrated. Weeks 32–37 I was in Labor and Delivery for contractions at least once a week. I couldn't keep down enough water to make them stop. I had my daughter at 38 weeks.

Originally, my husband and I wanted to have at least three kids. Now, I feel like we will be lucky to have just two. When (or if) I get pregnant again, if I have HG again, it will be the last time. Working was a nightmare. I have a wonderful boss and good insurance coverage. Still with insurance, my medical bills ended up being over $3000. I am still paying them off. I could barely work part-time when I was pregnant. Especially my first trimester. I couldn't ride/drive in a car without hurling. When I was pregnant, I hated hearing, "it'll all be over soon" or "it'll all be worth it in the end." I just wanted to die. But, it was true. My little girl was very much worth it. I envied everyone who had a "normal" pregnancy. I wanted so bad to be excited for my baby and to be glowing and fat and happy. Instead, I was hungry, sick, and miserable. I was starving all the time, but too sick and scared to eat anything. I can't even say how many nights I spent curled up on the floor in the bathroom. I was lucky to have understanding doctors, although it was hard trying to explain to everyone else why I was so sick. Everyone had their own cures and advice and I wanted to tell them to "shove it!"

Kelsy

I found out I had Hyperemesis at 7 weeks of pregnancy. Before that, every time I went to the doctors, my keytones were always high. I was so dehydrated—losing so much weight. Being Type1 diabetic my blood sugars were so low due to the fact that I couldn't keep anything down.

Finally, one time while I was getting fluids, my doctor told me I would need to go to the hospital because nothing they were doing was really helping and they needed to get me medicated. So to the hospital I went and that is when I was seven weeks and found out I had Hyperemesis. They put me on Reglan and Zofran and I tell you after the third day I was able to eat and drink again WITHOUT throwing up. This was a major improvement to the previous two weeks. I actually thought I was cured when I left. They had me taking the pill version of Zofran and Reglan by my fourth day and discharched me on the fifth because I was taking so well to it.

Well on the sixth day back home, the vomiting started again—and being the complete hard head I was—this occurred at work. Yes, I went straight back to work after the hospital. I couldn't eat anything that week except soup, and the doctor put me off the vitamins. That Sunday I lost the soup too. Had to go back to the doctor on Monday and found out that my keytones were high and I was severely dehydrated losing over ten pounds that week.

So this time I am in the hospital for two weeks. This time I am vomiting while I had the IV and when they tried to get me to eat. The hospital tray would set it off. I had never been as sick as I was those two weeks. I remembered to my dismay just wising it could be over—wishing that the pregnancy would terminate. I thought I was dying. I felt like I was dying. I thought I was going to lose my job and my husband would stress me out about the finances with two hospital visits. No one really understood. People told me I just needed to get up cut my hair, and do something during the day. All I wanted to do was lay there—I had no energy from the vomiting to even move. I looked like a heroin addict at this point. My lips peeling, my hair matty,—only thing I could bare to do with myself was take a shower and that was severe because it would cause me to throw up. Well, on the day I was discharged I still couldn't keep anything down and my doctor told me I just needed to take a shower and I would feel better after I told him how sick I was feeling that morning already. Well, needless to say, three days later I'm right back where I started in the ER severely dehydrated.

I was on short term disability approaching my 14th week—trying in vain to eat anything—then one day on my 15th week I noticed I was able to eat chicken noodle soup and grits!!!!!!! So morning would be grits and lunch and dinner chicken noodle soups—this is all that I have consisted of since 14 weeks. I am also able to drink hot tea (that really helps with the nausea at times) and at times water late at night before I go to bed. Don't forget the ice cream; I can also eat that usually before I go to bed.

I am now 17 weeks and the worst of the nausea has moved up towards 4:00 to about 9:00 whereas two weeks ago it was all day. Today I had a breakthrough and was able to eat a hamburger—without the bun—bread makes me sick.

I am now able to keep weight steady, I haven't gained and I haven't lost. I am still not eating the calorie intake my doctor would want me to—and I still look horrible due to the dehydration. I think I just have to take it one day at a time and eventually it will pan out.

I'm working again from home and doing the best I can—eating the best I can. I still have my ups and downs but hoping as the weeks go on, the ups will be better than the downs.

It is nice to know someone is writing a book about this. I wish I had found a book on it when I was first sick—it's always nice to know you're not alone in this hell.

Testimonies for Caregivers

I would like to share something that I learned in the early stage of HG. Sometimes it's just OK. It's OK if I need to cook. It's OK that she doesn't do the laundry. It's ok that she doesn't feel well because I'm sure that if she had a choice this is not the way she would choose to feel. It's OK if she goes and lies down. It's all going to be OK.

There is more I would like t share. That feeling you get when your wife cries and begs for your help. It shows how much you desire to help. I hope that feeling never goes away. The simple truth is all you can do is hold their hair; hand them a wash cloth; and tell her you love her from the bottom of your heart, and you are there for them.

I'm sorry that we can't do more.

Neil

We've been living the nightmare of HG for five weeks now. If there is anything I can offer from our experience, it's that you, dad, have to be the advocate. You have to demand better care. Your wife is so sick she can hardly think straight, let alone stand up to a doctor. You can't allow her to be lost in the medical system.

Force your doctor into action. Don't assume that just because your doctor is an experienced OB that he knows any more about HG than you do. Make your doctor become educated. If he won't, find a new OB.

Don't assume that your doctor knows anything about what is going on with you. Despite the growing availability of electronic charting, the doctor probably didn't check the chart before he called you. He probably doesn't know that his partner gave you four liters of fluid when he was off yesterday.

The messages that you leave for your doctor rarely make it to him intact. What you say is filtered back to you. If you suspect your doctor isn't getting the whole picture, fight your way through the blockade that the nurses put up and speak directly to the doctor.

Don't let an inexperienced nurse stick your wife. An HG woman isn't somebody to practice starting an IV on. If it isn't started on the second stick, get somebody else. Find out who the best nurse or phlebotomist in the hospital is and get them to do the stick. If you have an outpatient cancer care center, the nurses there are likely to be good with needles.

Get a referral to a perintologist, a specialist in maternal-fetal medicine. They have likely seen more cases of severe HG and should know or be willing to learn about more aggressive treatment options. We finally saw one and he had all kinds of options for us, far more than the three things our OB tried.

Don't be afraid to call your hospital's patient advocate. They have ways of getting things done. If you're afraid of retribution by your OB, get a new one.

Patrick
First time Dad

1. http://www.Kroger.com/HN_HOMEO/What_Is_Homeopathy_hm.htm

2. http://www.sosmorningsickness.com/whocanhelp.html

3. http://www.mo-river.net/health/coping_nausea.htm

4. http://www.morningwell.co.uk/tpm.htm

5. http://www.wellnessex.com/nausea_or_morning_sicknessis%20Grav …

6. http://www.hyperemesis.orguk/homeopathy.htm

7. http://www.gentlebirth.org/archives/earl/.jpg

8. http://www.helpher.org/hyperemesis-gravidarum/treatments/index.php

9. http://www.thefurrymonkey.co.uk/picc.htm

10. http://www.theparentsite.com/pregnancy/smoothie.asp

11. http://www.netrition.com/cgi/healthnotes.cgi?contentID=1046004

12. http://www.gingerpeople.com/recpe_pancakes.html

13. http://pub75.ezboard.com/fchefmomcomfrm49.showmessage?topicID=26.topic

14. http://atoz.ighealth.com/HealthAnswers/encyclopedia/HMLfiles/3017.html

15. http://www.kroger.com/HN_Homeo/Morning_sickness_hm.htm

16. http://clos.net/lib/04_comps/nausea/steroids.htm

17. http://qjmed.oxfordjournals.org/cgi/content/abstract/89/2/103

18. http://qjmed.oxfordjournals.org/cgi/content/full/95/3/153

19. http://www.moondragon.org/obgyn/pregnancy/morningsickness.html

20. http://www.Gynob.com/morningsick.htm

21. http://www.findarticles.com/p/articles/mi_MOCYD/is_20_37/ai

22. http://www.helper.org/hyperemesis-gravidarum/treatments/nutritional-therapy/parenteral- …

978-0-595-44200-3
0-595-44200-5

Printed in Great Britain
by Amazon.co.uk, Ltd.,
Marston Gate.